The Female Reproductive System

Penguin Library of Nursing

General Editor
Michael Bowman

The Cardiovascular System
The Digestive System
The Endocrine System
The Female Reproductive System
The Neuromuscular System
The Respiratory System
The Skeletal System
The Urological System
The Special Senses

The Penguin Library of Nursing Series was created by
Penguin Education and is published by Churchill Livingstone.

C. N. Hudson

The Female
Reproductive System

Churchill Livingstone

CHURCHILL LIVINGSTONE
Medical Division of Longman Group Limited

Distributed in the United States of America by
Longman Inc., 19 West 44th Street, New York,
N.Y. 10036 and by associated companies,
branches and representatives throughout
the world.

First published 1978

ISBN 0 443 01609 7

Library of Congress Cataloging in Publication Data

Hudson, Christopher N.
    The female reproductive system.

    (Penguin library of nursing)
    Bibliography: p.
    Includes index.
    1. Gynecologic nursing. 2. Generative organs,
Female—Diseases. 3. Generative organs, Female.
I. Title. [DNLM: 1. Reproduction—Nursing texts.
2. Gynecology—Nursing texts. 3. Obstetrics—
Nursing texts. WY157 H886f]
RG105.H8   618'.1   76-53016

Printed in Great Britain by
Richard Clay (The Chaucer Press) Ltd,
Bungay, Suffolk

Contents

Editorial foreword

Nursing has undergone considerable change during the past decade. There have been many developments in medical science and technology, and nursing education must keep pace with these changes, not merely in principle, but in terms of the nurse's attitude and approach. These changes primarily stem from the move towards caring for the patient in the context of his entire personality – the concept of total patient care. This concept was originally underlined in the 1962 Experimental Syllabus of Training and has subsequently been mirrored with greater emphasis in the 1969 Syllabus.

The education of the nurse, as voiced nationally and professionally in this decade, has merited prominence; this is certainly underlined in the recent *Report of the Committee on Nursing* (Briggs). It now appears likely that the once rather mythical education of the nurse is now approaching reality and fulfilment. For too long there has been conflict between the service needs of the hospital and the education of the nurse.

These require effective marriage if student satisfaction and general job satisfaction of the officers concerned and, perhaps most important of all, good patient care are all to be achieved. It is hoped that this series of textbooks will go some way towards helping students achieve a better understanding, in a more interesting way, of what this concept of total patient care is all about.

The series consists of nine books; together, these books make up an integrated whole, although each can be used in isolation. Each book embraces developmental embryology, applied anatomy and physiology, pathology, treatment, nursing care, social aspects and rehabilitation of the patient. In addition, each book contains a comprehensive list of further reading for the nurse.

It is hoped that students will find much pleasure in reading these books.

Michael Bowman
Principal, Education Division, Hendon Group Training School
Examiner to the General Nursing Council for England and Wales

Preface

It is almost presumptuous for a doctor to write about nursing care, and this work could not have been attempted without the advice and criticism afforded by my nursing colleagues, Miss Hazel Champion and Miss Elizabeth Capper.

The role of the nurse in the gynaecological ward is a very special one, physically not usually very heavy but often emotionally taxing. On occasions the success of operations is totally dependent on the postoperative nursing care. It is a pleasure to record my gratitude to the nursing staff of our gynaecological unit who have inspired the content of this book by their consistently high standards. I am grateful too to Miss Susan Hales who drafted the illustrations and to Mrs Caryl Hudson who typed the text.

C. N. Hudson

Chapter 1   Introduction

Gynaecology is the medical speciality concerned with the female organs of reproduction. In some places this term covers disorders of the breast, but this is not universal. Symptoms related to the organs of reproduction rank high amongst complaints which may cause a woman to visit her doctor. Consequently, in hospital practice gynaecological surgery occupies an important place in the work of the hospital, and only too often the waiting lists are depressingly long. The importance of the subject to the nurse, however, does not merely stem from the volume of work performed in gynaecological departments.

The role of the nurse

The very nature of the work means that the nurse often has a special part to play in the management of patients with this type of complaint.

The patients coming into the gynaecological wards are often frightened about the impending operation or treatment, unsure of its implications and rather hesitant to ask for further explanation. Many patients remember little of what they were told in the clinic and need a sympathetic, informed nurse to listen to their problems and to outline the proposed treatment, explaining what it will involve and how they will feel afterwards; listening is as important as speaking. Often they are busy women with heavy household or professional responsibilities who need help to unwind, then enjoy the enforced rest. Many are worried about their families, especially where there are young children involved, and it may be necessary to enlist the help of the Medical Social Worker if no one can be found to care for them. Later it is necessary to give some guidance as to the amount of activity recommended during the convalescent period and when they can resume normal work.

The interplay of patients' responses is very noticeable in gynaecology. In a strange way, there is a great sense of kinship amongst them, women who have only just met will quickly be exchanging detailed medical and family histories. It happens too, that if one patient becomes emotionally distressed, others in the ward are also likely to become so. It is important for the nurse to remember this, so that she is tactful and patient, even under stress. As in most wards, the patients will listen with great interest to anything that is said to any one of them. The nurse needs to be sensitive to this, particularly when carrying out intimate procedures, endeavouring to avoid embarrassment to her patient. Many patients have a natural reservation about such intimate matters, and it may well be that they feel more able to unburden themselves to a sympathetic nurse than, perhaps, a doctor. Moreover, some patients may talk to a nurse about bodily functions related to these organs without making a specific complaint. The nurse may thus be in a privileged and rather special position in that she can perhaps appreciate the significance of symptoms of which a woman speaks. Urgent advice to seek medical opinion may be necessary. This may well happen in general medical or surgical wards and can be of considerable importance both to the patient and to the doctor. A nurse should be well acquainted with the range of normal function in these organs, and also with the significance of abnormal symptoms. Moreover, it will be useful to her to be familiar with the side-effects and results of various treatments.

Patients will sometimes talk about their marital problems to the nurse and frequently confide their fears about fulfilling their role as women postoperatively. Problems can sometimes arise if the nurse is not particularly careful when counselling the patient, especially on the resumption of sexual intercourse, as the patient may be recently widowed or an elderly spinster or in the process of separation or divorce and can easily be upset or offended.

Conflict of aims can arise for the student nurse when she finds herself nursing patients anxious to have a baby and those having a pregnancy terminated in the same ward. An understanding of both their needs is required, and care should be taken to keep such patients separated.

Old wives' tales

No branch of medicine is more bedevilled by folklore and hearsay than that relating to the female genital tract, and there can be very few patients who come into hospital for a gynaecological operation who have not in some way or another been 'brain-washed' by well-meaning friends or relatives. The nurse should be familiar with the popular misconceptions about gynaecological procedures so that she may anticipate her patient's fears and anxieties and be in a position to allay some of them.

Development and evolution of the female genital tract

Many *vertebrates* (animals with backbones) reproduce by laying eggs. The most highly developed of the vertebrates are the *mammals*. A mammal is an animal which suckles its young at the breast, and the majority belong to the group called *placental animals*. These grow their young inside a muscular organ called the *uterus* or womb until they are of sufficient size and maturity to have an independent existence after they are born.

Nearly all female mammals have intermittent episodes of sexual activity known as *oestrus* or being 'in season' or 'on heat'. At these times they will receive the male but not, usually, at other times. During oestrus there is a blood-stained discharge from the female parts, as anyone who has kept domestic pets will know.

The human female, in company with certain higher apes, is unusual in that she does not have episodes of sexual activity, but will receive the male at all times during the reproductive years of her existence and for many years afterwards. In this special group of higher mammals (the *primates*) the loss of blood at monthly intervals, which is commonly referred to as 'a period' or *menstruation*, is not to be confused with the oestrus which occurs in the rest of the mammalian world. At oestrus, the vaginal loss is associated with ovulation, whereas menstruation is the discharge of blood mixed with the lining of the uterus (womb) which had been prepared following ovulation about a fortnight earlier for a pregnancy which has not taken place. After menstruation is over a fresh lining develops growing from the basal cells of the glands which have been preserved, and the whole process is repeated again at monthly intervals unless pregnancy supervenes.

Reproduction

The bodies of all higher animals consist of multitudes of small units which are known as cells. The process of reproduction consists of the fusion of one special *germ cell* (*gamete*) with another from an individual of the opposite sex. The fused cell (the *zygote*) then divides again and again, eventually growing into a new individual.

The fusion of two gametes brings about a 'shuffling' of inherited characteristics from either parent. The mechanism of this 'shuffling' is a reduction by half of the genetic material or *genes* in each cell during the production of gametes. Each gamete will have a different distribution of genes. Fusion restores the quantity of genetic material to the normal level for the cells of the new individual, but the genes come equally from the two parents.

Because the genetic material is distributed differently in individual gametes, brothers and sisters who are not identical twins will differ from each other in many ways, although they may share some general characteristics.

The female genital organs

We will now consider the general arrangement of the various organs of reproduction and the way in which they work. The major components are the *ovaries*, the *uterus* (the womb), the *oviducts* (Fallopian tubes), the *vagina* and the *vulva* (Figure 1). The detailed anatomy and physiology of these organs will be considered in later chapters.

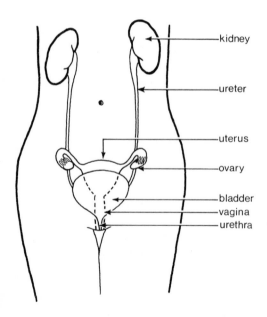

Figure 1 The female genito-urinary system

Table 1 Functions of the female genital organs

Copulation	Sexual intercourse
Ovulation	The formation and liberation of 'egg cells' or 'oöcytes' (formerly called ova)
Conception	The beginning of a pregnancy considered in two phases:
Fertilization:	the union of a germ cell from a male partner with the female oöcyte to form a zygote
Implantation:	the embedding of the zygote in the wall of the uterus
Menstruation	The discharge of blood and cellular debris from the uterus when a pregnancy has not been established

The ovaries

The oöcytes (ova) develop within paired structures known as the *ovaries*. The ovary is the female counterpart of the testis but in contrast to the male, the female gonad is entirely abdominal and lies within the peritoneal cavity. It also has a very much firmer consistency than the testis and feels almost hard to the touch.

This hardness is due to the fibrous texture of the ovarian substance (*stroma*). Within this stroma are to be found microscopic cysts which develop into *Graäfian follicles* containing the ripening oöcytes. Although the oöcytes are laid down very early in development, long before birth, they do not begin to ripen until puberty, which marks the beginning of the reproductive era.

The uterus

The ovary may be likened to a factory which produces the seeds of reproduction, and the *uterus* can be similarly compared to a seed bed where a new plant will sprout from the tiny seed which has been buried in the lining wall. The uterus of the human female is usually a pear-shaped midline muscular structure occupying the middle part of the bony pelvic basin. The muscular wall (the *myometrium*) is thick, consisting of unstriped muscle not under voluntary control. The main part of the uterus is called the body or *corpus*. The lower narrow part or neck is a fibro-muscular ring called the *cervix*.

The oviducts (Fallopian tubes)

Stretching from either corner (*cornu*) of the uterus towards the ovary is a thin-walled muscular tube called the *oviduct*. Each oviduct is somewhat similar in size to the appendix and, like the uterus, each is covered with a shiny membrane of peritoneum, except at the end where the lining ceases abruptly at the *fimbriated portion*. Here the tube has an open mouth ringed by a series of tassels (*fimbriae*) which give it an appearance reminiscent of a sea anemone.

The oviducts capture and transport the oöcytes, which are discharged free from the ovary into the general peritoneal cavity. Unless a discharged oöcyte is picked up by an oviduct and transmitted towards the uterus, the whole process of reproduction will fail. During this transit the act of fertilization occurs, before the oöcyte reaches the cavity of the uterus.

The vagina

Below the uterus is a muscular skin-lined tube which is approximately 8 cm long and which is flattened under normal conditions, the front and back walls being in contact with each other. This tube, the *vagina* is named from the Latin word meaning a scabbard or sheath. There is elastic tissue as well as muscle in the wall of the vagina, which is capable of considerable stretching to allow the passage of a baby during childbirth.

The *cervix* known colloquially as the 'neck of the womb' projects into the upper part of the vagina; it is usually closed but, like the vagina, is capable of considerable expansion during childbirth.

The vulva

The *vulva* is the area of skin which surrounds the lower end of the vagina. It consists of two lips (*labia*) on each side and the phallus which, in the female, is called the *clitoris*. The skin of the labia is specialized and corresponds to that which forms the scrotum in the male. The clitoris, like the male penis, is erectile but the *urethra* (the tube carrying urine from the bladder) is separate and discharges within the vulva onto the area known as the vestibule, which lies below the clitoris.

Development of the female genital organs

In both sexes special germ cells develop very early and become grouped in organs called *gonads*. In the male, the gonad, called *testis* or testicle, descends from a position high up in the abdomen right down to the scrotum. In the female, a similar descent is interrupted in the pelvis but the blood supply to the ovary is derived from the region of the kidney in just the same way. In the male, the duct of the primitive kidney is adapted for use in adult life as the vas deferens which carries the spermatozoa (the male germ cells). This duct becomes vestigial in the female but may occasionally give rise to cysts alongside the vagina, known as Gaërtner's cysts.

The female genital tract develops alongside the duct of this primitive kidney as a duct which is known as the *paramesonephric* (or Müllerian) duct. It is a paired organ and the two ducts give rise to the oviducts, which fuse to form the uterus and upper portion of the vagina.

Errors of development

Variations in the development of these two paramesonephric (Müllerian) ducts give rise to a number of congenital abnormalities of the female genital tract. One duct may be totally absent or vestigial, giving rise to a uterus which has only one oviduct attached to it and only one cornu or horn (*unicornuate uterus*). Degrees of failure of fusion may lead to several varieties of reduplication of the lower genital tract.

Complete reduplication leads to a *double uterus* with double cervix and two separate vaginae. One side of this duplicated genital tract may be less well-developed than the other and this can be a considerable source of diagnostic confusion. Lesser degrees of duplication occur in which there is a single uterus containing two separate cavities, or a cavity with a partial septum (wall) between the two upper parts. These minor abnormalities of the uterus may have little effect upon reproductive ability but can be of obstetric importance because they can alter the position which the baby takes up in late pregnancy and cause unfavourable conditions for natural childbirth.

The adult kidney develops at much the same time as the adult genital tract and it is not, therefore, surprising that those patients with a congenital abnormality of the female genital tract show an increased incidence of abnormalities of the urinary tract. One important anomaly involves a *ureter* (the tube leading from the kidney to the bladder) opening into the vagina or urethra. Such an *ectopic ureter* (Figure 2) represents either an accessory ureter or a misplaced normal ureter.

It seems that the female structure in human beings represents the basic structure and that the male form is evoked by special hormones (see p. 21) produced by the male gonad. If there are serious disorders in the genetic material, the proper differentation of sex may not occur. When this happens the gonad will fail to develop altogether and in the adult will be represented by a streak of white fibrous material; one condition

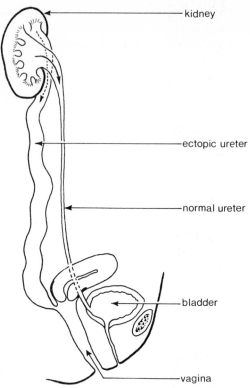

Figure 2 Ectopic ureter opening into the vagina. Note the dilatation of the abnormal ureter due to obstruction and infection

in which this occurs is known as *Turner's syndrome*. Sometimes the paramesonephric ducts fail to develop on both sides and there is then total failure of development of the internal genitalia. Both these two extremes of congenital abnormality may present with the symptom of failure of the onset of menstruation (a condition known as *primary amenorrhoea*).

At one stage in its development, the vagina is quite solid, and canalization occurs later. If there is failure of completion of canalization the same symptom of primary amenorrhoea may occur but, in effect, menstruation may well be occurring above the dam of the incompletely canalized vagina. This means that month by month a small collection of altered blood forms in the space of the vagina, getting bigger and bigger as time goes by. The periods in this instance are not absent but hidden and the term *cryptomenorrhoea* is applied. Sooner or later it becomes a matter of urgency that the way to the exterior be opened up to allow menstruation to occur in the normal fashion. The condition is often referred to as an imperforate hymen and the retention of menstrual fluid is called *haematocolpos*.

Summary of nursing points

The role of the female genital system must be understood in the context of the woman's physiology and psychology. The nurse must understand the development, structure, functions and role of the system as a whole. She must appreciate that the disorders of this system may have social and psychological effects on the patient which may be of a transient or permanent nature. In this context the nurse must be sensitive to ensure privacy and do all she can to minimize any embarrassment during such intimate procedures as gynaecological examination, vulval toilet, catheterization and pubic and vulval shaves.

Chapter 2   Ovulation, copulation and menstruation

Ovulation

Germ cells for the subsequent generation can be identified in the
gonads at a very early stage in development. During the reproductive
years in those mammals which have a menstrual (as opposed to
oestrous) cycle, the oöcytes (ova) are shed at intervals into the
peritoneal cavity in a process known as *ovulation*. This is one point in a
regular monthly cycle (Figure 3) which involves the pituitary gland

changes in the ovary

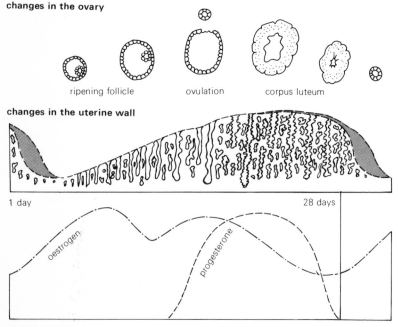

ripening follicle   ovulation   corpus luteum

changes in the uterine wall

1 day   28 days

oestrogen   progesterone

changes in hormone levels

Figure 3 The ovulatory cycle

(located at the base of the brain, above the roof of the mouth), the ovary and the lining of the uterus (the *endometrium*). Each month, following menstruation, special substances are released from the pituitary gland at the base of the brain into the blood stream. These substances, which act as chemical messengers, are called *hormones* and they produce a definite physiological action in so-called 'target' organs in distant parts of the body, where there are cells particularly sensitive to such substances. In this instance the pituitary gland produces a hormone which is known as *follicle stimulating hormone* (FSH), and its production is regulated from the adjacent area of brain, known as the hypothalamus, by the production of a *releasing factor*.

The action of FSH is to cause one Graäfian follicle (see p. 15) containing an oöcyte to ripen. It is not completely understood why all the follicles in the ovary do not ripen at once. If several follicles were to ripen simultaneously, there would be a distinct possibility of multiple pregnancies occurring. Follicle stimulating hormone may be used as treatment for certain forms of infertility, when there is a failure of ovulation. It seems that the dose used may be critical in determining the number of follicles which ripen and this is the reason for some of the dramatic multiple pregnancies which were notorious in the early days of treatment of what has been known as 'anovulatory infertility'.

As the follicle ripens, it in turn produces its own hormone from the outer rim of cells known as granulosa and theca cells. These hormones also circulate in the blood and are known as *oestrogens*. There are several different varieties, all of which act on the uterus and other parts of the body, such as the breasts. The uterine effect is one of the most important, and is characterized by an additional ripening process, this time of the endometrium. In this oestrogenic phase the endometrial glands proliferate and grow, thus becoming tortuous and convoluted, hence the name *proliferative phase*.

As the cycle progresses, the pituitary gland produces another hormone, known as a *luteinizing hormone* (LH). Both these hormones from the pituitary are given the generic name of gonadotrophins (the suffix 'trophin' usually implies a substance which promotes or nourishes a specific organ). Luteinizing hormone is so-called because it is responsible for the production of a body in the ovary known as the *corpus luteum* ('yellow body'). It is this luteinizing hormone which is largely responsible for ovulation. There is a very significant surge in the output of luteinizing hormone some hours before the rupture of the ripening follicle through the cortex of the ovary. When the follicle actually ruptures, the oöcyte is discharged into the peritoneal cavity and it is those cells remaining on the outside of the follicle which take on a yellow appearance and are called the corpus luteum. At this time the hormone production changes and, while oestrogens continue to be produced, an additional hormone, *progesterone*, with different pharmacological actions is also produced (see Figure 3).

Whereas oestrogens promote rapid growth of the glands and proliferation of the cells of the endometrium, progesterone slows down the division and multiplication of cells so that they mature and take on functions which they could not develop during the phase of rapid division. The maturing endometrial cells are said to be in the *secretory phase*, and the glands become much more convoluted and begin to secrete. One other hormone from the pituitary is particularly concerned with ovulation. This is prolactin, but, unlike the other gonadotrophins, it is elevated levels of prolactin which suppress ovulation.
In the event that pregnancy does not occur, menstruation will ensue, and the cycle will start again.

Copulation

Fertilization is the direct result of *sexual intercourse* (also known as *coitus* or *copulation*). The act of copulation requires the insertion of the erect male phallus into the vagina. If this is attempted too quickly, it can be a difficult and painful procedure; so the act of penetration and copulation is usually a sequel to a period of courtship and preliminary preparation which enables the female genital tract to become suitably receptive. In the female the phallus is a small organ (the clitoris) situated in the anterior part of the vulva, over which the two labia minora form a hood (see p. 80). The clitoris is capable of erection just as the male phallus is, and it is responsible for much of the sensation of sexual activity, although, in the female, the breasts play an important role as areas of sexual activity.

The vagina is normally lined only by stratified squamous epithelium similar to skin and does not contain glands. There are, however, a group of glands (notably Bartholin's glands, see p. 83) at the vulva which produce their secretion at times of sexual activity. They discharge into the vestibule via ducts in the region of the hymen. The position of the ducts is of some importance, as they may be injured in lacerations or incisions at the time of childbirth. With adequate courtship or foreplay, the secondary sexual organs of the female are brought to a state of readiness so that, when penetration occurs in the act of copulation, rhythmic activity may be set up resulting in a climax which is known as an orgasm.

In the male, orgasm is associated with ejaculation of the seminal fluid, which will be deposited in the upper end of the vagina. In the female, orgasm is not such a discretely identifiable moment and it is important to realize that an orgasm in the female is not essential for conception as it is in the male. It is important to realize, too, that even penetration of the vagina is not absolutely necessary for conception. If the male ejaculates somewhere near the lower end of the vagina, sperms can travel up it and bring about fertilization if other circumstances are favourable. The fact that a girl is still a virgin is not therefore an absolute bar to her becoming pregnant. The term virgin implies that the hymen, which is a partial membrane across the lower vagina, has not been ruptured. Such rupture must occur on the first occasion that full penetration occurs during intercourse and this may be responsible for some bleeding and pain. The aperture may be stretched digitally beforehand, and this may have been done to facilitate the insertion of tampons for the control of menstrual flow.

Copulation is not confined to the reproductive years and may continue long past the time when fertility has ceased.

The social implications of sexual intercourse do not need elaboration. Within a marriage or stable union the ability to copulate with satisfaction may be fundamental. Lack of interest in sexual activity (loss of libido, *frigidity*) is a common complaint and may be the underlying factor behind a woman's gynaecological complaints. The apparent presenting symptoms may be an imagined or real excuse for avoiding intercourse and the husband may have persuaded the woman to seek medical advice.

It may not be enough to establish that loss of libido is the real basis for the complaint. It is necessary to go further and look for the antecedent cause. The side-effects of the contraceptive pill should be recognized, as well as a suppressed fear of pregnancy. Perhaps the most important and most common cause is depressive illness. This may be endogenous, but can be secondary to the *climacteric* (change of life, see p. 32) and —to a delayed and sometimes unrecognized reaction to pregnancy (*puerperal depression*). The total change of family environment caused by the intrusion of the first baby and the disruption of social life which it entails can have a profound influence on the emotions and relationship between husband and wife. This may be a difficult time too for the professional woman who has to give up or curtail her job. Those who devote themselves entirely to being wives and mothers may feel the disappointment from 'opting out' when the children are suddenly grown and leave home.

Gynaecological conditions which cause pain or interfere mechanically with intercourse have implications far beyond their medical importance. This is particularly relevant to complications of surgery for perineal lacerations at childbirth or for vaginal prolapse (see p. 100). In developing countries, native medicine men find the vagina a convenient receptacle for their potions and, if the patient survives the immediate severe complications which may include heavy metal poisoning and renal failure, the end result may be impenetrable stricture.

Fertilization

During the reproductive years, whenever the male ejaculates in the vagina some 2 to 3 ml of his seminal fluid are deposited in the upper vagina near the cervix. This male fluid contains many million spermatozoa or 'sperms', the reproductive cells which are the exact equivalent of the female oöcyte. These cells are extremely small, consisting mostly of nuclear material, but they have a long tail which renders them motile. The swarm of sperms ascends through the cervical canal and then over the endometrium right up the fundus of the uterus (Figure 4). They swarm along the oviducts and, if the time of the cycle is right, will there meet the discharged oöcyte which has entered the tube from the peritoneal cavity. There the act of fertilization occurs.

It only requires one sperm to penetrate the capsule of the oöcyte for nuclear fusion to occur, thus bringing about the union of the two 'half-sets' of genetic material (see p. 13), but it seems that a large number must be present to enable this one to get through. Possibly this is because semen contains an enzyme (hyaluronidase) which may facilitate the breaking of the cell membrane of the oöcyte.

Once the oöcyte has been fertilized, it moves slowly on down the Fallopian tube (Figure 5) and, immediately, the nuclear material starts to divide so that what was one large cell soon becomes a bunch of small cells. This bunch, called the *morula*, soon develops a central cavity and

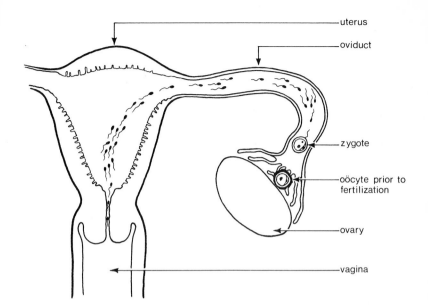

Figure 4 Pathway of fertilizing sperms

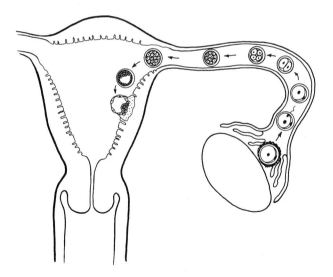

Figure 5 Path of zygote (fertilized ovum). Note how cells divide

at this stage is termed the *blastocyst*. There is very early differentiation within the blastocyst of two distinct areas – the *embryo* goes on to become the definitive individual of the next generation, while the *trophoblast* is responsible for establishing the connection between the embryo and the mother. The trophoblast gives rise, in due course, to the placenta, cord and membranes. These are passed after the birth of a baby.

Implantation

At this stage, the trophoblast consists of two layers of actively dividing cells which have properties of invasion very similar to those possessed by malignant cancer cells. When the blastocyst arrives in the

Blastocyst   **Implantation of trophoblast**

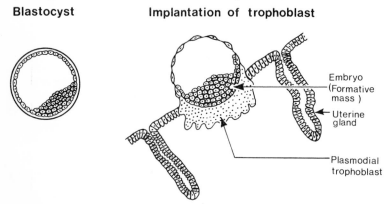

Embryo
(Formative
mass)

Uterine
gland

Plasmodial
trophoblast

Figure 6 Implantation of the blastocyst. The trophoblastic cells invade the endometrium

endometrial cavity, the trophoblast very quickly penetrates the surface of the secretory endometrium (Figure 6), so that the whole small embryo rapidly becomes buried within the endometrium. The time interval between fertilization and this process of *implantation* may be about a week. There are, therefore, only a few days left before the next menstrual cycle is due to occur. This corresponds to a time when the pituitary gonadotrophins FSH and LH are withdrawn as a result of direct suppression of the pituitary, sometimes referred to as a 'feedback' mechanism. Unless something occurs to replace these hormones, the corpus luteum will fail and, in turn, the oestrogens and progesterone which maintain the endometrium in its lush state will also be withdrawn. Spasm of the vessels and infarction will occur, resulting in sloughing of the endometrium and the onset of a menstrual period. A tiny blastocyst hidden in this shed endometrium would be lost to the outside world without anyone being aware of its existence.

For successful pregnancy to occur, this menstrual period must therefore be postponed and some vital phsyiological activity must thus take place quite rapidly following the time of implantation of the zygote (fertilized ovum). This activity is one of the functions of the trophoblast. In theory the trophoblast could either undertake the immediate production of oestrogens and progesterone, or it could produce gonadotrophins similar in action to FSH and LH. Although the trophoblast later becomes a most important producer of ovarian steroids, at this stage it is incapable of producing sufficient for the purpose and instead it produces a gonadotrophin and thus maintains the existing 'factory' for oestrogens and progesterone, namely the corpus luteum. The gonadotrophin which is produced is given the name *chorionic gonadotrophin* after the layer of the trophoblast from which it is produced.

Human chorionic gonadotrophin (HCG) is produced very early in pregnancy, as indeed it must be in order to maintain the corpus luteum. Its production rises to a peak at three months and then tails off to be present in varying quantities for the remainder of the pregnancy. It is a substance which is excreted in the urine and its detection, therefore, is the basis for the modern tests for pregnancy. Chorionic gonadotrophin is so similar to luteinizing hormone (LH) that very few tests will distinguish between the two, and it is only the large quantities of HCG which are present in pregnancy which are regarded as diagnostic of pregnancy. Occasionally, however, in older patients the levels of luteinizing hormone may be sufficiently high to render one of the standard pregnancy tests positive. There are rare conditions other than pregnancy which can cause the presence of chorionic gonadotrophin in the urine, so it is important to realize that pregnancy tests are not strictly tests for pregnancy, but only for chorionic gonadotrophin.

Development of the fetus and placenta

Once the menstrual period which is due shortly after implantation has been suppressed, the trophoblast soon undertakes the production of its own oestrogens and progesterone in increasing amounts until the end of pregnancy. Thus it very rapidly becomes independent of the corpus luteum, which may be removed without harm to the pregnancy. The trophoblast at this stage consists of a shell round the blastocyst covered with fine processes which are known as *chorionic villi*. Very soon the

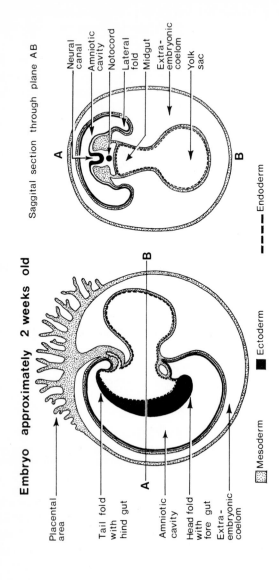

Figure 7 Development of the fetus

Approximately 3 weeks old

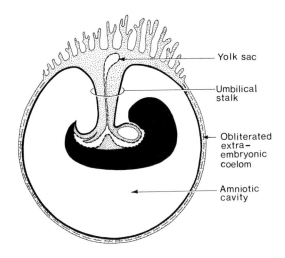

Yolk sac

Umbilical stalk

Obliterated extra- embryonic coelom

Amniotic cavity

Figure 7 Continued

villi disappear from most of this surrounding shell, leaving a smooth area called *chorion laeve*. The shaggy villi remain concentrated in one area near the base, known as the *chorion frondosum*.

As the embryo (Figure 7) develops into a recognizable human being, a primitive heart is formed and circulation begins. Certain blood vessels develop very early, namely the arteries of the primitive bladder and the veins of the primitive intestine. Both these structures have part of their development outside the actual embryo and become connected up with capillaries which form in the centre of each chorionic villus. As the baby (now called a fetus) develops, a leash of vessels from the chorion frondosum become twisted together in a cord called the *umbilical cord*. Within the chorion is another layer of membrane called the *amnion*, within which there is free fluid surrounding the fetus.

The fetus is connected by the umbilical cord to the chorion frondosum, which is later given the name *placenta* and forms a 'plate-like' structure in intimate contact with the endometrium; so intimate, in fact, that the chorionic villi actually erode into the maternal blood vessels. These villi are bathed in a pool of maternal blood which allows the exchange of waste products and nutrients between the baby and the mother.

The baby, therefore, has developed a system for being a perfect parasite. As a parasite it is able to grow and exist at the expense of the mother. On the other hand, it is not subjected to the reactions which human tissues would normally show to those of another individual of unlike genetic make-up. These reactions (*immune reactions*) are responsible for the rejection of skin grafts and other tissue grafts from different individuals. In pregnancy, however, the placenta constitutes an immunological barrier against rejection of the developing fetus. This barrier is not absolute and, under certain conditions, harmful immunological responses in the mother can, in fact, reach the baby, particularly if there is discrepancy in the blood group known as the Rhesus factor.

The further consideration of the progress of pregnancy and parturition is beyond the scope of this book, but disorders of early pregnancy are regarded as lying within the field of gynaecology, and patients who suffer from them are usually nursed in gynaecological wards.

Menstruation

This discussion has considered the physiological events which may follow the event of copulation, namely conception, fertilization and implantation. It remains to consider what occurs if this chain of events does not take place. In any menstrual cycle when pregnancy does not occur and after an average interval of 28 days, a further menstrual period will occur. Earlier it was stated that immediately following a menstrual period activity of the pituitary gland produces hormones which lead to ripening of a follicle. Ovulation in response to a surge of such hormones occurs with rupture of the follicle and discharge of the oöcyte into the peritoneal cavity.

The remains of the follicle forming the corpus luteum are responsible for the production of ovarian steroid hormones, the oestrogens and progesterone, which in turn have two effects which are of importance to the cycle. First they stimulate the proliferation of endometrium and then, by slowing down the process, allow the endometrium to mature and enter what is called the secretory phase. At the same time, both the ovarian hormones have a feedback effect via the hypothalamus upon the pituitary gland, depressing the production of the pituitary gonadotrophins. These gonadotrophins are then withdrawn and this reduces the activity of the corpus luteum and, hence, the production of ovarian hormones.

At this point, in the absence of a pregnancy with its own gonadotrophins, the oestrogens and progesterone are withdrawn and the endometrium which has been built up under their influence is no longer able to survive. The blood vessels go into spasms and dilate again, and haemorrhage occurs into the endometrium causing infarction and sloughing. This brings about the classical and monthly loss of blood known as menstruation. Characteristically this blood does not clot, as the uterus is able to produce an anti-clotting agent. If, however, the loss is heavier than normal clots may well occur as there will be insufficient of this agent to prevent their formation. Clots are a definite sign that a period is abnormal (see p. 38).

It is important to realize that menstruation represents the end of a cycle and that the bleeding is entirely different from the blood-stained discharge of oestrus which occurs at or around the time of ovulation in other animals. Very occasionally, ovulation can occur at times other than in mid-cycle and may perhaps be provoked by intercourse. A pregnancy has been known to occur from isolated acts of intercourse at the end of a menstrual period.

Menstruation usually occurs at approximately monthly intervals from the early teenage years until approximately 50 years. The onset of menstruation is a feature of the development of secondary sexual characteristics which is known in both sexes as puberty, and this onset is called the *menarche*.

The menopause

The cessation of periods is likewise called the *menopause*. It is important to realize that this normally occurs in three well-defined ways – the periods may finish abruptly without any warning, the periods may remain regular and get less and less in quantity, or they may get further and further apart until they finish. There may be a combination of the last two ways. *Any other variation in menstruation at the time when the menopause may be expected is not normal.* Irregularity of menstruation at this time is not particularly uncommon but must be regarded as pathological and occasionally of serious import. It is vital, therefore, that this irregularity of menstruation be regarded as a symptom for which medical advice should be sought.

This is the sort of situation where a nurse may be of paramount assistance to a patient who may never have complained of abnormal menstruation, but may confess to a nurse who is looking after her that her periods are behaving in this way. A nurse who recognizes that this pattern can sometimes be the presenting symptom of a serious disease and can advise the patient to seek appropriate advice will be doing a great service. Apart from the cessation of periods around the age of 50, other symptoms may occur at this time of life, some of which may be attributable to the alteration in the hormone pattern.

This episode in a woman's life is correctly referred to as the *climacteric* rather than the menopause, which is a term which should be reserved strictly for the cessation of menstruation. Symptoms occurring at the time of the climacteric are variable and some of them are unrelated to the actual occurrence of the menopause. Nevertheless, there is a considerable folklore associated with the so-called 'change of life' and many patients are offered gratuitous and well meaning, but ill-informed, advice on symptoms which occur at this time. A tendency to ascribe all ills and depressions at this time to the climacteric is certainly to be deprecated, and can be responsible for patients failing to seek advice and treatment about unrelated important conditions.

Effects of menstruation

The cyclical hormone changes produce profound effects on the internal environment and the alteration of mood, ability to concentrate and general performance are well recognized. This may be of considerable importance to a woman in a professional position and its relation to important events such as examinations is obvious. In the same context, the symptom of dysmenorrhoea (see p. 95) can give rise to considerable disability and, although a well-recognized phenomenon, may be a factor in the commercial world where loss of time from work is involved. Disorders of menstruation assume greater importance if a woman is single or the breadwinner, and treatment may be determined by a particular necessity to a patient to go back to work as soon as possible. This is not to say that menstrual disturbances are not important to the housewife, but the timing may not be so crucial. For any woman, the chronic ill health induced by excessive menstruation is not always reflected by an overt degree of anaemia, and should not be judged by this alone.

Social embarrassment caused by flooding can be acute and, once experienced, can keep a woman confined to the home whenever she is at risk.

Summary of nursing points

The nurse must understand how hormones work and where they are produced, and the important role they play in the menstrual cycle. It is wise to consider the menstrual cycle as three cycles in one: the pituitary cycle, the ovarian cycle and the uterine cycle.

The student must appreciate the problems associated with puberty, both physiological and psychological, and be capable of advising the young girl on such problems in an effort to reduce and obviate anxiety, bewilderment and apprehension. She must also be able to recognize as abnormal events attributed by the patient to the menopause.

Chapter 3

Disorders of the uterus and menstruation

Disorders of the uterus and disorders of menstruation inevitably form a major part of gynaecological practice. In many developing countries, however, there is a traditional reluctance to admit to any disorder of menstruation for fear that the uterus may be removed. In Caucasian communities, women are not so inclined to put up with the inconvenience and discomforts of abnormal menstruation and will, by contrast, seek medical advice for such symptoms. The implication is that they will accept the advice necessary for treatment even if, on occasions, this means removal of the uterus.

Anatomy of the uterus

The uterus is a pear-shaped organ situated above the vagina, above and behind the bladder and in front of the upper part of the rectum. It consists of a body (*corpus*) expanded at the top where the two oviducts enter (Figure 8). That part of the uterus situated just above the entrance of the tubes is called the *fundus* and the lowest part, the neck, which projects into the vagina is called the *cervix*. The vaginal surface of the cervix is lined with a covering of epithelium similar to skin, but its canal is lined by glandular epithelium which secretes mucus.

The internal lining of the uterus lies directly on the thick muscular wall called *myometrium* (Figure 9). Contractions of this muscular wall occur during the process of childbirth or labour and expel the baby through the cervix, which must dilate before the baby can pass down the vagina and be born. These contractions can occur and cause pain at other times, such as during abortion or even sometimes during menstrual periods. The pain is to be likened to cramp and is similar to colic which may be felt from the intestine. The immediate cause of uterine contractions may be the local release of substances called *prostaglandins*.

Before puberty the uterus is quite small; it enlarges greatly during pregnancy and regresses to a small size again after the menopause. The

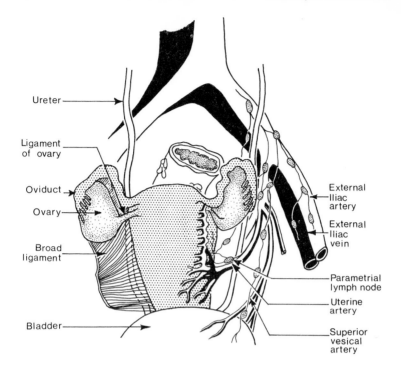

Ureter

Ligament of ovary

Oviduct

Ovary

Broad ligament

Bladder

External Iliac artery

External Iliac vein

Parametrial lymph node

Uterine artery

Superior vesical artery

Figure 8 The uterus, showing the blood supply

process of shrinking after childbirth is known as *involution*.

The outer surface of the body of the uterus is covered by the glistening membrane of peritoneum (see Figure 9) and thus projects free in the peritoneal cavity within the 'basin' of the pelvic cavity. Only when enlarged, as by pregnancy or tumour, will the uterus rise into the abdominal cavity where it can then be detected by palpation.

The peritoneum is firmly attached to the underlying myometrium and cannot be readily stripped. It is reflected off the front of the uterus on to the dome of the bladder. In this region the peritoneal attachment is loose, as the bladder is an organ which requires to fill and empty at intervals and needs space in which to expand. The loose attachment of the peritoneum to the front of the uterus allows the bladder to use the potential space in this region.

The peritoneum is reflected as a double sheet from each oviduct to

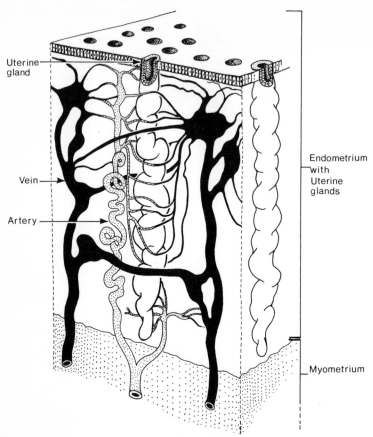

Uterine gland

Vein

Artery

Endometrium with Uterine glands

Myometrium

Figure 9 The blood supply to the uterine wall. All the arteries supplying the endometrium have to traverse the muscular wall (the myometrium)

form a structure called the *broad ligament* – not really a ligament at all, but a fold of peritoneum. Near the insertion of each oviduct is attached a cord-like structure which is also encased within the broad ligament. This is called the *round ligament* and is attached to the anterior abdominal wall in the region of the inguinal canal. This ligament helps keep the uterus angled forwards on the vagina (anteversion). Laterally, the broad ligament contains loose connective tissue known as the *parametrium*.

The cervix is covered by peritoneum in its upper part only at the back. The peritoneum is then reflected off to form the lowest part of the peritoneal sac of the pelvis which is called the pouch of Douglas. In the front the cervix is intimately related to the bladder and it is not surprising that disorders of either of these may affect the other. On occasions this can lead to diagnostic confusion and to a lesser extent, this can also apply to the large intestine behind. Inflammatory conditions in the pelvis can cause the intestine to adhere strongly to the back of the uterus and indeed collections of pus in the pelvis can 'point' into the upper vagina. The proximity of the bladder base to the cervix means that the terminal portions of the ureters are very close to the side of the cervix and must always be in the thoughts of a gynaecological surgeon operating in this area.

Abnormal menstruation

Normal menstruation consists of a vaginal haemorrhage occurring in a cycle of roughly a month. There is, however, nothing magic about 28 days and variation of a few days on either side of this is perfectly acceptable. If the cycle of menstruation becomes reduced so that the interval between the first day of any period and the first day of the subsequent period is of the order of 3 weeks or less, then the term *polymenorrhoea* is used. It is slightly confusing that the term *oligomenorrhoea* is used to describe both a loss which occurs at normal intervals, but is of smaller quantity than usual, and a markedly prolonged cycle. Frequently, however, such a scanty loss is associated with a prolonged cycle.

Continuing this terminology, the term *amenorrhoea* is used to describe absence of menstruation. This, of course, is a normal situation at certain times. Before puberty (that is to say, during childhood) and after the menopause, amenorrhoea is normal. If menstruation never starts, the term *primary amenorrhoea* is used (see p. 18). Amenorrhoea is also the rule during episodes of pregnancy and is common after pregnancy while breast feeding is occurring. Amenorrhoea which sets in some time after the onset of menstruation (the menarche) is called *secondary amenorrhoea*. Apart from pregnancy, secondary amenorrhoea may be due to hormonal imbalance, sometimes secondary to emotional and environmental stress and at other times to a definite pathological condition, such as tuberculosis. It is a symptom, therefore, for which a patient should seek skilled medical advice if it persists for more than a few months. In particular, advice should be sought if there are associated complaints, such as infertility or increase in the amount of body hair (*hirsuties*).

Painful menstruation is known as *dysmenorrhoea* and will be considered in Chapter 6.

Heavy menstrual bleeding is referred to as *menorrhagia* and, strictly speaking, this should be entirely regular. It is difficult to lay down objective standards whereby heavy menstruation may be judged, but the passage of clots and the use of more than two dozen sanitary towels is usually regarded as good evidence that the loss is considerably more than average. There is no set termininology for irregular bleeding except that an episode of prolonged bleeding, lasting more than 10 days, is referred to as *metrorrhagia*.

Irregular bleeding is a very important symptom as it may be due to cancer of the uterus, so all patients with this complaint should seek medical advice. This is one situation where a nurse may offer unsolicited advice to *any* patient she is looking after, should she become aware that the patient is suffering from irregular vaginal bleeding.

Investigations of menstrual abnormality

Cervical cytology

Cells which are shed from the endometrium may lie in a small collection in the posterior fold (fornix) of the vagina and can be collected on a wooden spatula which is inserted for this purpose. More important, however, the surface cells of the cervix can be scraped off by such a spatula and likewise smeared on to a glass slide. This procedure is known as taking a *smear*, a phrase which is widely understood by members of the public. It is a procedure with which a nurse should be fully familiar. In some situations a nurse may be trained to take smears herself.

Instruments required:
    bivalve speculum
    Ayre's spatula
    glass slide
    marking pencil
    fixative solution.

Procedure

The speculum is inserted with the patient lying on her left side, and is opened to expose the cervix. The tip of the Ayre's spatula (Figure 10) is inserted into the external aperture (*external os*) of the cervix and rotated through 360 degrees. Both sides are immediately smeared

bivalve speculum

Ayre's spatula

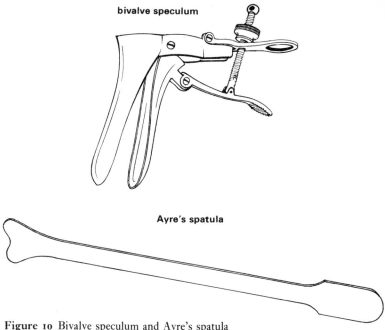

Figure 10 Bivalve speculum and Ayre's spatula

all over one surface of a glass slide and then the pool of mucus in the posterior fornix (see p. 69) is picked up with the other end of the spatula and similarly smeared on to another slide. Both slides must be liberally sprayed with fixative solution *before* they have dried. Sometimes the fixative is supplied in pots into which the slides must be dipped, or in dropper bottles, in which case the slide must be flooded. Once the slides are fixed, they should be allowed to dry, and can be sent through the post for staining or taken to the laboratory without undue haste.

The exfoliated cells when stained by the method of Papanicolaou (often called 'Pap' stain for short) can give information about a variety of conditions. The cells from the vagina will show variations according to the type and time of the menstrual cycle and may also show evidence of inflammation, especially due to *Trichomonas vaginalis* and *Candida albicans* (see Ch. 5). The smear from the cervix will very accurately demonstrate the presence of malignant cells from a cancer of this region. The cells from the posterior fornix pool have approximately a

50 per cent chance of showing evidence of cancer of the endometrium. By implication, this means that 50 per cent of patients with this type of cancer are not diagnosed by smear, and this in turn means that all patients potentially at risk will require a further diagnostic test.

Dilatation and curettage

This very common minor procedure (*D and C*) is largely of diagnostic value. It consists of *dilatation* of the cervix with a series of graduated rods until it is sufficiently open to admit the passage of small sponge-holding forceps and a spoon-like scraping device known as a *curette*.

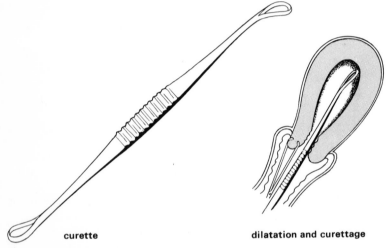

curette   dilatation and curettage

Figure 11 Dilatation and curettage

With this equipment the cavity of the uterus may be explored (Figure 11) and polyps (see p. 42) and so forth removed, together with the endometrium which may be scraped off.

All material obtained in this way will be placed in formalin and sent for histological examination, except in instances where the diagnosis of tuberculosis is suspected, when part of the curettings must be preserved in saline and not formalin. The specimen will be used for the bacteriological culture of the *Tubercle bacilli*. It is important for the nurse who is working in an operating theatre to appreciate this distinction because, once curettings have been placed in formol-saline, they are useless for bacteriological culture. Both these specimens will require careful labelling and an appropriate laboratory request form.

Treatment of menstrual abnormalities

The diagnostic procedures outlined above are normally coupled with careful physical examination, which may be made much easier by the use of anaesthetic. They will be necessary to exclude malignant disease in the first instance, and to determine the size, shape and mobility of the uterus together with an assessment of the ovaries and tubes (sometimes called the appendages or adnexa).

The definitive treatment may be dictated either by the underlying condition or, if this is not determined, by the symptoms of the patient.

1 In the absence of organic disease, the curettage alone may bring about relief of symptoms in a small proportion of patients, even though it is performed for diagnostic purposes.

2 Certain types of hormone imbalance may be recognized, and the use of hormonal substances, colloquially known as 'the pill', is one form of treatment for this type of menstrual disturbance. This form of treatment is quite acceptable in youngish women, but is better avoided when the menopause is approaching.

3 A small dose of deep X-rays used to produce an irradiation artificial menopause has an occasional place in the treatment of abnormal periods when the natural menopause is imminent. Radium insertions are no longer used for this purpose.

4 Usually, however, for patients for whom child-bearing is no longer anticipated, the operation of simple total hysterectomy is to be preferred. This avoids the unpleasant physiological effects of an artificial menopause and at the same time removes the source of the bleeding and any further worries about contraception. The effects and side-effects of hysterectomy need to be understood in some detail by a nurse, and will be considered later in the chapter (p. 47).

Structural causes of menstrual disturbance

Fibroids

The most important structural (organic) cause of disturbed periods is a benign condition called *fibroids* (Figure 12). These are fibromuscular tumours of the uterine muscular wall. They are extremely common, affecting approximately one woman in three during her lifespan, and are almost entirely benign. The symptoms that fibroids produce are related to the actual site in which they may be found.

Subserous fibroids jut out from the uterus into the general peritoneal

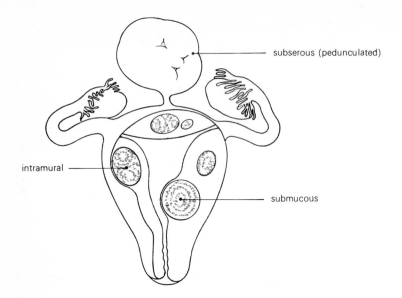

Figure 12 Fibroids

cavity and may produce symptoms from their sheer size or from the possibility of disturbance to their blood supply by torsion or other forms of infarction. They may be a source of diagnostic confusion to gynaecologists, as their distinction from solid tumours of the ovary may be difficult. Subserous fibroids do not, as a rule, provoke disturbance of menstruation but they may press on the bladder or bowel.

Intramural fibroids lie within the wall of the uterus and cause distortion of its shape, which is one of the diagnostic features. Often, but not always, they provoke disturbance of menstruation by causing enlargement and distortion of the endometrial cavity. They may cause pressure effects in the same way that subserous fibroids do.

Submucous fibroids are really subendometrial in position and project into the uterine cavity. They may occasionally be extruded through the cervix on a pedicle, in which case they will be responsible for prolonged blood-stained discharge, sometimes sufficient to cause profound anaemia. At other times, they must inevitably cause disturbance of menstruation.

Cancer of the uterus

The other main organic cause of disturbance of menstruation is cancer of the uterus. In many instances this will present as bleeding after the menopause (so-called 'postmenopausal bleeding'), but in a significant number of cases the presentation will be at, or well before, the natural cessation of periods. There are two main sites, the cervix and the endometrium, and the behaviour of growths in these two areas is quite different.

Cancer of the endometrium

This tends to occur in the older age group of patients, but about one-fifth of these cases will still present before the menopause. It does, moreover, have a tendency to be associated with infertility or small families. There is an added association with obesity and diabetes mellitus. Cancer of the endometrium remains confined to the uterus for a long time and presents early due to its bleeding. It is, therefore, amenable to surgical treatment, which consists of removal of the uterus and both ovaries. Some centres will use radiotherapy in addition either before or after the operation and rarely is the disease disseminated. Additional treatment with progesterone-like hormones can be of value.

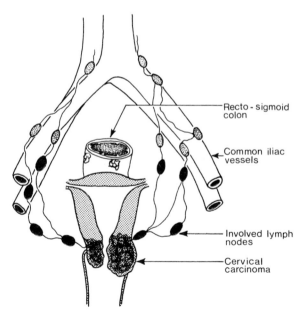

Figure 13 Lymphatic spread of cervical cancer

Cancer of the cervix

This is a disease of much more sinister import which tends to afflict the younger age group of patients, the majority being in the 40–50 age group. The disease spreads more rapidly than cancer of the endometrium and soon involves the lymph nodes (Figure 13) in the pelvis on either side. Eventually the disease spreads forwards and backwards to involve the bladder and the rectum, so that it is quite possible for a patient to end up with a double fistula, urine and faeces leaking through the vagina. The latter may be alleviated by a diverting colostomy, but the former presents formidable problems in management. It is particularly distressing when this occurs in a relatively young woman with a growing family, and a young nurse faced with a patient in this situation may feel it keenly. The implications of the disease go deep, because the maximum incidence of cancer of the cervix is during the later child-bearing years when the woman may have a young and growing family which is very dependent on her. Cancer of the cervix is a disorder of sexually active women, and there is an association with early onset of sexual activity and with promiscuity involving a number of sexual partners.

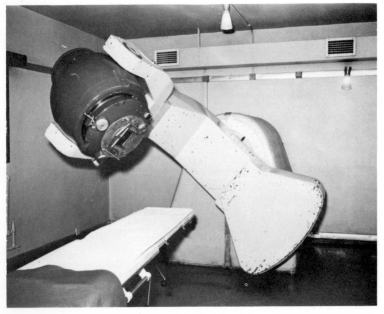

Figure 14 Cobalt bomb

The standard treatment of cancer of the cervix is radiotherapy. In most instances this consists of local application of a radioactive substance, usually caesium, in a tube, which may go inside the cervical canal, and in either boxes or ovoids which are placed in the vagina and held in place by a special applicator. Following insertion of these radioactive sources, most patients are treated, in addition, with external therapy using high-voltage apparatus – often the 'cobalt bomb' (Figure 14).

From the nursing point of view, gynaecological radiotherapy requires certain definite precautions. The removal of the radioactive pellet may

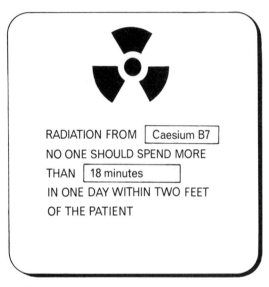

RADIATION FROM Caesium B7
NO ONE SHOULD SPEND MORE
THAN 18 minutes
IN ONE DAY WITHIN TWO FEET
OF THE PATIENT

Figure 15 Labelling used at foot of bed of patient receiving radiotherapy

occasionally devolve upon the nursing staff and this has to be carried out at an exact time after the insertion. All patients who have radioactive material within them have to be nursed with special precautions, including the display of a suitable warning notice (Figure 15), and keeping a lead-lined box near the bed. Sometimes this is carried out in a separate radiation ward, but in gynaecological hospitals the radium or caesium patients are frequently nursed in the open ward. In nearly all hospitals there is a Radiation Safety Officer, and the nurse should know how to contact him.

It is very important for the nurses in the ward to be fully acquainted

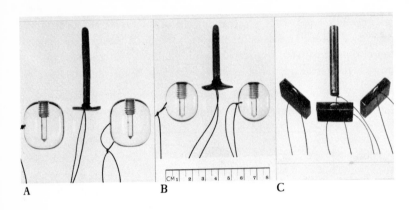

A   B   C

Figure 16 A. Radium applicators for a Manchester insertion, large. B. Manchester insertion, small. C. Radium applicators for a Stockholm insertion. (*From* Howkins, J. and Hudson, C. N. *Shaw's Textbook of Operative Gynaecology*. 4th edition. Edinburgh: Churchill Livingstone.)

with the appearance of the sources (Figure 16) and of their dangerous nature; under no circumstances must a nurse pick these up by hand or put them in her pocket, or make any gesture of this sort. Occasionally the patient may pull out the packing and the sources herself while in a semiconscious or confused state as a result of the anaesthetic and, occasionally, also, the sources may be passed either into the bed or into a bedpan. It is part of nursing routine to count the threads attached to the sources every 8 hours while they are in place. For this reason, all patients who have radium in place should never be allowed to go to the lavatory, but must pass all excreta into a bedpan, and they will also normally be fitted with a self-retaining catheter so that micturition will present no problems unless the patient attempts to pull the catheter out. If the patient is in a general ward, pregnant staff or visitors and patients in the child-bearing age group should be kept at a distance. Staff treating the patient should wear film monitors and modern units will supply a Geiger counter for checking irradiation contamination.

During the phase of external irradiation, patients may show signs of a general reaction. They may get diarrhoea and nausea and frequently become very depressed, so the maintenance of morale and general support from the nursing staff is extremely important for this type of therapy.

Finally, in some centres, radical surgery is still applied for cancer of the cervix, the operation is known as Wertheim's radical hysterectomy, and may be combined with radiotherapy.

Abdominal operations on the uterus

Preoperative preparation

Practice will vary from unit to unit, but most surgeons will require skin preparation and removal of hair from the pubic region and lower abdomen, either by clipping or shaving. Pelvic operations are always more difficult if the bowel is loaded, but postoperative wind may well be aggravated by enemata. A modern practice is to make sure that the bowel is empty by means of the insertion of suppositories.

Some important investigations are carried out before almost all gynaecological operations, and the Ward Sister will want to see that the results have been returned to the notes. These results include the haemoglobin level, the blood group, chest X-ray and cervical smear. In malignant disease it may also be necessary to perform an *intravenous pyelogram* (in this examination, a radio–opaque dye is injected into a vein; the dye will normally be concentrated by the kidneys and passed into the urine, and X-ray photographs of the kidney region will reveal any structural abnormalities).

Otherwise the preparation and premedication is the same as for any major abdominal operation. This includes routine ward testing of urine for sugar and protein, baths using bactericidal soap, and persuading the patient to increase her fluid intake right up to the time when preoperative starvation begins. It is usual for the patient to have a sedative to help her sleep the night before. The usual consent forms are required but, in many units where the operation of hysterectomy is contemplated, it is the custom to have the consent form countersigned by the husband, as it is an operation which is going to procure sterilization.

If the woman is pregnant the green form required by the Abortion Act (see Ch. 8) must have been signed.

The nurse has a very important role to play in allaying unspoken fears and anxieties which the patient may be keeping to herself. The patient should be encouraged to talk about these beforehand because they are so often founded upon misconceptions which have been acquired from well meaning but ill-informed friends. This discussion should form part of the routine when explanation of the operation is given at the time of signing the consent form.

The operations

Incisions for gynaecological operations are either vertical (in or near the mid-line) or transverse. The latter are becoming more popular and are sometimes called Pfannenstiel incisions.

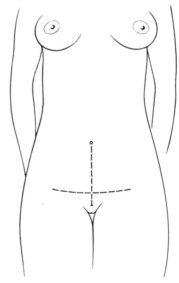

Figure 17 Laparotomy incisions

Myomectomy

This is the simple enucleation of fibroids from the uterus, which is then sewn up. This operation is performed through a standard laparotomy incision (Figure 17).

Total hysterectomy

This is the commonest operation for benign conditions and it is often useful to describe this procedure to patients as a removal of 'that part of the womb which is responsible for bleeding'. It is not what is commonly referred to as the operation for 'taking it all away'. It involves, in fact, removal of the body and cervix of the uterus but, in its simple form, the tubes and ovaries on both sides and the entire length of the vagina are left intact (Figure 18). As far as the patient is concerned, this operation has two effects, and two effects only. First, there will be no more periods and, secondly, there will be no more pregnancies. There are no other effects of total hysterectomy, whatever 'old wives' tales' may attribute to this operation.

More extended operations

Hysterectomy with additional bilateral salpingo-oöphorectomy

The removal of both appendages (Figure 18) extends the operation of total hysterectomy and is sometimes referred to as a *pan-hysterectomy*. It is carried out when diseases of the ovaries or oviducts are present (such as cysts or tumours) and as part of most operations for cancer. Inevitably this extension of the operation involves the production of a surgical menopause unless it is carried out on a patient who has already passed the menopause, when it adds nothing to the postoperative symptoms. Indeed this addition is usual in patients who have passed the menopause, as generally they are having their operation for some disorder of the ovaries or tubes.

Radical (Wertheim's) hysterectomy

This is the operation of 'taking it all away'. It consists of removal of the uterus and appendages, the upper one-third (at least) of the vagina and a wide expanse of tissue on either side (the broad ligament and parametrium, see p. 50), together with the lymph nodes which lie in the region of the major iliac vessels on either side of the pelvis. (Figure 18). There are, of course, individual variations in the extent of the operation, but basically this is common to all of them. In contrast to simple total hysterectomy, radical hysterectomy leaves a large raw area in the pelvis which may be covered with peritoneum, but nevertheless the potential dead space for haematoma formation is very much greater.

An extensive Wertheim operation may have two unwelcome long-term consequences associated with the interference in the act of micturition. The extensive lateral dissection may well damage the parasympathetic motor nerve supply to the bladder producing paralysis of the detrusor muscle (the bladder muscle). The patient, therefore, may have considerable difficulty in emptying the bladder afterwards and readily goes into 'overflow incontinence' (in which the bladder is so full of residual urine that any more arriving from the kidney immediately

Standard total hysterectomy

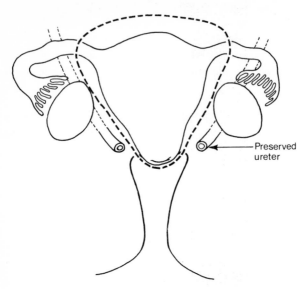

Preserved ureter

Radical (Wertheim's) hysterectomy

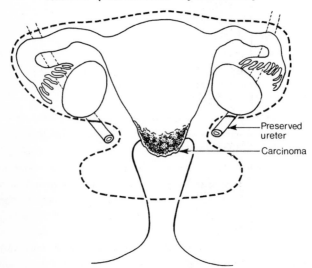

Preserved ureter

Carcinoma

Figure 18 Extent of tissue removed in different types of hysterectomy operation

Extended total hysterectomy & bilateral salpingo-oöphorectomy

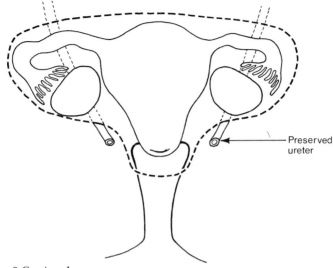

Preserved
ureter

Figure 18 Continued

overflows). Additionally, she may suffer from an infected residual urine. Furthermore, the extensive mobilization and removal of vagina may well interfere with the support of the bladder-neck closing mechanism and provoke the onset of severe stress incontinence (see p. 106) which is very difficult to deal with.

Postoperative nursing and complications

The immediate complications of any major abdominal operation are shock, haemorrhage and sepsis. It is important to remember in gynaecological operations that there are two wounds: one easily visible on the abdominal wall, the other within the vaginal vault. Primary haemorrhage, when it occurs, may visibly discharge from the vagina into the bed and, as part of the immediate postoperative observation of a patient, inspection of the pads to determine the extent of the vaginal loss is a vital part of nursing care. It is, however, also possible for bleeding to occur inside the abdomen above any pack which may be present in the vagina, so that signs of internal haemorrhage may develop without outward evidence of bleeding. Therefore regular nursing observations on the vital signs of pulse rate and blood pressure are particularly important, as these may give the first clue to internal bleeding.

The other vital signs to be observed during the first 24 hours while the patient recovers from anaesthetic are complexion and respiration, with particular attention to the airway. In addition, to the vulval pad, drainage sites and dressings should be inspected.

The nurse will be responsible for maintenance of any intravenous infusion and changing the bottles as required. Occasionally the patient may return from the operating theatre with an epidural catheter in place, and this may be used to provide postoperative pain relief. Otherwise the nurse is responsible for anticipating postoperative pain and nausea with timely exhibition of sufficiently powerful analgesics and anti-emetics. When she has recovered consciousness, the patient will appreciate a gentle wash and the return of false teeth and so forth. Care and attention to the small details of patient care at this time are an integral part of good nursing. Attention to a patient's position is, however, more important than a matter of mere comfort, as the development of pressure sores and venous thrombosis can be related.

During the postoperative period the nurse must pay particular attention to the patient's urine output. Patients who have had extensive operations will have an in-dwelling catheter (Figure 19), but this is not usual with the ordinary total hysterectomy. A few of these patients do have difficulty in passing urine after an abdominal operation in which, rather naturally, the back of the bladder has suffered some bruising in the course of the manipulation to free it from the uterus. It is usual, however, to allow the best part of 12 hours before insisting that a catheter be passed on such a patient, and it is often reasonable to allow such a patient to use a bed-side commode which she may find easier. With a Wertheim's hysterectomy, however, an in-dwelling catheter is usually left in for at least a week, and sometimes longer.

There are special risks associated with gynaecological operations to the urinary tract and the ureters: the urethra or the bladder may suffer direct injury or necrosis (tissue death) as a result of interference with the blood supply (the latter is particularly likely in patients who have major cancer surgery and who have been treated with radiotherapy beforehand). Such injuries, if unrecognized at the time of operation, or if brought about after operation by necrosis, will result in the formation of a fistula with abnormal discharge of the urine or, if the bowel is involved, faeces from the vagina. The occurrence of a wet bed or pad may be the first outward sign that a mishap of this sort has occurred, and it is as well for the nurse who is in charge of the gynaecological

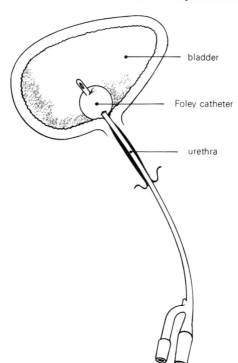

bladder

Foley catheter

urethra

Figure 19 Catheter draining the bladder

ward to be aware of this. If a patient appears to be incontinent after a major operation, the doctor should be informed at once because it may well be that the leak of fluid is not through the urethra, but from an abnormal fistulous communication.

It is equally important to note if urinary output is low or absent. This may be due to blockage or kinking of the catheter, but sometimes may be a sign of a more sinister complication; there may have been obstruction to the ureters during the course of the operation, and further surgery will surely be necessary. Alternatively, a patient who has been in surgical shock for any length of time may develop acute renal failure, which needs early diagnosis and treatment. If intravenous fluids continue to be administered as usual to such a patient, she may literally drown in her own internal fluid. Mixtures containing potassium salts are particularly dangerous at this time – these include fruit juices and the ubiquitous 'Mist.Pot.Cit'.

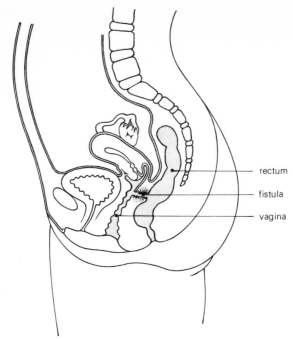

rectum

fistula

vagina

Figure 20 Rectovaginal fistula

It may sometimes be difficult to determine the difference between the discharge of the contents of a pelvic abscess from the vagina and the development of a faecal fistula (Figure 20), but a complaint by the patient of the passage of wind through the vagina is highly suggestive and, eventually, if there is anything other than the smallest fistula, faecal matter will readily be identified.

Following operations on the genital area, patients may usually eat and drink earlier than they would in a general surgical ward after abdominal operations but, of course, the complication of paralytic ileus may possibly occur, so that distension and vomiting should be viewed with suspicion, and oral feeding should not be forced under these circumstances. A major complaint of patients following pelvic surgery is distension with wind and, as soon as the wind begins to pass freely through the rectum, their discomfort will be at an end.

The problems of wind seem less with early administration of oral fluids (usually the same day as the operation) and light diet (usually started the following day). Early mobilization also helps, and patients are often encouraged to sit out of bed and even take a short walk on the day following the operation. The problem usually resolves itself when the bowels open and, to aid this, a suppository is often given on the third day.

With modern waterproof dressings, patients are allowed into a bath well before the sutures are removed. It is very important that the nurse (*not* the patient) should be responsible for disinfecting the bath before and after use. A patient who is a little unsteady will be glad of assistance at this time. A patient will not be allowed into the bath until packs and drains have been removed, and it is considerate to give an analgesic injection prior to such removal or indeed any other treatment which could cause distress. This is not necessary for the removal of clips or sutures, for which there will be a local routine; this may be delayed for a variety of reasons such as obesity, diabetes or cancer.

The occurrence of diarrhoea after a few days, particular in the presence of a raised temperature, is suggestive of irritation of the bowel by a collection of blood which may have been infected – the so-called infected *pelvic haematoma* or pelvic abscess. This will usually clear itself at 10 to 14 days by the discharge of material, which has been likened to anchovy sauce, or possibly even frank pus from the vagina; the patient should be warned that this is likely to happen and not to be alarmed. A certain amount of blood-stained discharge from the vagina is common and may go on for quite some time. It is, however, rare for frank secondary haemorrhage to occur. When it does, it should be treated seriously and may require that the patient be taken back to the theatre to have the bleeding point sealed either by suture or packing. The ordinary postoperative discharge requires regular vulval toilet before bathing is established.

Normally after hysterectomy a patient is ready to go home by about 10 or 11 days. Such an operation will take more out of a patient than perhaps she realizes, and it is usual to arrange convalescence. Women often do not find it easy to rest once they get home because many are expected to run the family, and it is one of the duties of the nursing staff to acquaint the relatives with the fact that the patient will require care and attention and relief from housewifely burdens for some weeks following her discharge from hospital.

It is important too, to talk about the resumption of sexual relations to these patients. Many will be concerned about this but will have been too shy to talk about it. After the standard total hysterectomy, reassurance can be given that there will be no interference with intercourse. This reassurance, however, cannot be given with a radical Wertheim's hysterectomy because the vagina will have been made very much shorter by this procedure, and it is better for the doctor to explain the problems which may ensue and what can be done to alleviate them. It is important, however, to make sure that the patient and her husband realize that there is a fresh wound at the top of the vagina and that, if intercourse is resumed immediately on going home, disruption of the vault may occur resulting in a severe secondary haemorrhage and injury. It is best that intercourse should be forbidden for some three months, until the patient has been seen by the doctor and an examination has proved that all is well-healed.

Some patients will feel acutely that they have lost their femininity by having a hysterectomy. There are no grounds for this apprehension at all in patients who have only had the ordinary total hysterectomy and whose ovaries have been conserved. Nevertheless, although much less marked than in patients who have had breast operations, a feeling of having been mutilated may be present, and should be understood. The emotional reactions of a childless woman are readily understandable, as hysterectomy irrevocably destroys any unfulfilled dream of potential reproduction, however unlikely this may have been up to the time of operation. These patients will need particular psychological support after the operation, and a skilled nurse will recognize the appropriate approach for each individual patient.

Summary of nursing points

As disorders of menstruation are the most important evidence of uterine disorders, the nurse must acquaint herself with the causes, signs and symptoms – and acquire the knowledge of how to support the patient physically, socially and emotionally.

The main conditions affecting the uterus are fibroids and carcinoma. The nurse must understand the usual forms of medical and surgical treatment for these. If treatment is surgical, then pre- and postoperative care is of paramount importance; preoperative care includes assessment of the patient's general health, observing blood pressure, pulse, temperature, respirations, urine and bowels and reporting any abnormalities. After the operation, the nurse must look for signs of haemorrhage or the presence of shock, observe the degree and nature of any pain and care for the wound, bladder, bowels and drainage. In addition, she must ensure that all drugs are given as prescribed, that the patient carries out the breathing and limb exercises necessary to prevent chest infection and venous thrombosis, and that the fluid balance is recorded accurately. As soon as permitted, the nurse must support the patient during mobilization and early ambulation. Finally, the patient must be counselled and supported socially and emotionally, particularly after very major surgery, which may have a depressing effect on her.

Chapter 4

Disorders of the ovary and oviducts

The ovaries and tubes are considered together because their functions are intimately connected, and any conditions of one usually involve the other. The *oviduct* is derived from the upper part of the primitive Müllerian duct system (see p. 17) which fuses together at the lower end to form the uterus and the upper part of the vagina.

Anatomy of the ovary and oviducts

Each *oviduct* is attached at its innermost end to the cornu (see p. 15) of the uterus. Indeed the lumen of the tube extends through the wall of the uterus and is continuous with the uterine cavity, this portion being referred to as *interstitial* or *intramural*. The rest of the tube is invested by the peritoneum of the broad ligament, the narrow part near the uterus being called the *isthmic portion* (not to be confused with the isthmus in the uterus, which is the intermediate zone between the body and the cervix) and the free, wider portion towards the other end being referred to as the *ampulla*. The open end is termed *fimbriated* because it is ringed by tassels (fimbriae) which give it an appearance like a sea-anemone. The tube is lined by a convoluted epithelium with intricate folds. The cells are cubical and have very fine hairs which help to waft the oöcyte down to the cavity of the uterus.

The *ovary* is likewise a bilateral structure, in size and shape somewhat similar to an unshelled almond. The surface is corrugated and the texture almost hard, in contrast to the smooth and relatively soft male gonad, the testis. Unlike the testis, the ovary is always an intra-abdominal organ, and is situated just below the oviduct on the back of the broad ligament. The ovary is tethered to the cornu of the uterus by the ovarian ligament and derives its blood supply from vessels which have their origin high in the abdomen near the kidneys. These vessels reach the ovary beneath the posterior leaf of the broad ligament and they branch to link with the uterine vessels, which come up from deep in the pelvis alongside the vagina and cervix.

Ovarian cysts

The ovary is developed from a structure in the embryo called the *germinal ridge*, which lies adjacent to the paramesonephric (Müllerian) duct system. It is not surprising therefore that certain cysts of the ovary may arise from cells similar to those from which the paramesonephric ducts arise. Indeed, formation of cysts is one of the most important features of pathology of the ovary. The smallest cysts in the ovary are not true new growths but are variations of the physiological cysts which form each month as part of the process of ripening the follicle.

If a ripening follicle fails to rupture, it may develop into a thin-walled smooth cyst called a *follicular cyst*. These rarely grow larger than about 3 cm in diameter. Occasionally, a corpus luteum may form a cyst called a *luteal cyst*. Finally, *multiple cysts (theca lutein cysts)* may arise as a result of excessive stimulation by a gonadotrophic hormone, either as a result of injudicious therapy in the treatment of infertility (see p. 65) or, more usually, because certain forms of abnormal pregnancy called vesicular mole (see p. 117), or an associated cancerous condition called choriocarcinoma (see p. 118), produce large quantities of chorionic gonadotrophin.

With these exceptions, cysts in the ovary should be regarded as new growths and, like all new growths, may generally be classed as benign or malignant. It is important, however, to appreciate the fact that there is an intermediate zone where the distinction between benign and malignant may not readily be drawn.

Many ovarian cysts have an internal lining similar to that of either the uterus, the cervix or the oviducts. The commonest are called *serous papilliferous cysts*. They contain a clear serous fluid and the inside of the cyst is filled with fine flower-like papillary fronds, which may occasionally penetrate to the outer surface of the cyst. The lining of these papilliferous cysts resembles that of the oviduct. Certain cysts are similarly lined with endometrium which may, like the endometrium in the uterus, undergo cyclical bleeding at the time of the periods and fill the cysts with altered blood. Such cysts are called endometrial or 'chocolate' cysts, and are part of a condition known as endometriosis, which will be discussed later (see p. 90). Finally, there are *mucinous* cysts (formerly called pseudomucinous) which are lined with tall, columnar mucus-secreting epithelium, very like the cells which line the glands of the endocervix.

Ovarian cancer

These three classes of cysts all have their malignant counterparts known as *serous papillary*, *endometrioid* and *mucinous cystadenocarcinoma* respectively.

Besides the common benign and malignant tumours of Müllerian origin, other tumours may arise from either the germ cells or the supporting stroma (fibrous tissue).

Stromal cell tumours

It is the supporting stroma cells which are responsible for the hormone production around the follicle, and it is not surprising that the cysts and tumours which arise from these may also produce hormones. The two important types are the oestrogen-producing tumours which are either called *granulosa cell carcinoma* or, if largely fibrous, *thecoma*. Many oestrogen-producing tumours contain both types of cell. Only the granulosa cell tumours may behave in a malignant fashion.

Occasionally, tumours of rather similar type and structure produce male hormones and the most important is called *androblastoma* (formerly called *arrhenoblastoma*). Sometimes a stromal cell tumour is entirely inactive, in which case it is very hard and called a *fibroma*. One special type of fibroma contains some islands of squamous cells and is known as a *Brenner tumour*.

Germ cell tumours

A tumour of germ cell origin usually contains several different varieties of cell and is known as a *teratoma*. Most teratomata in the ovary are benign and have a soft centre filled with pultaceous (pulpy) material and a solid area at one end which contains fairly well-differentiated tissue, such as bone, teeth, cartilage, salivary glands, sweat glands, skin and occasionally a variety of other tissues. This type of tumour is known as a benign cystic teratoma (colloquially called a 'dermoid' cyst, probably because one of its principal constituents is skin). A solid teratoma is much more rare and is usually malignant. Occasionally hormones may be produced by a solid teratoma, including chorionic gonadotrophin which can therefore give rise to a false positive pregnancy test (see p. 27). All of these tumours, particularly one called a *dysgerminoma*, are similar to tumours of the male testis.

Signs and symptoms

Ovarian tumours may grow to quite a large size before they give rise to symptoms, and huge growths bigger than a uterus at full term have been recorded. These may be quite painless, the obvious symptom being abdominal distension. If pain does occur, this may be a sinister sign, but it can be related to events such as haemorrhage into the centre of the cyst or leakage of the contents of the cyst into the abdominal cavity following rupture. If the cyst twists about its pedicle, then the blood supply becomes obstructed and infarction occurs. If the cyst thus becomes gangrenous, it will bring about an acute abdominal emergency requiring emergency surgery. If cysts do not present by abdominal distension or pain for the reasons outlined, pressure effects on neighbouring organs may give rise to symptoms. Vague sensations in the bowel and bladder may well be the only presenting feature of an ovarian cyst.

Ovarian cancer is not the most common cancer of the female genital tract, but it is responsible for more deaths in the United Kingdom than cancer in any other part of the genital tract. Its mortality now exceeds the combined death rate of cancer of both the cervix and the body of the uterus. There are several reasons for this depressingly high mortality. As with benign ovarian cysts, malignant tumours may well give rise to very few symptoms in the early stages and, indeed, in a high proportion of cases the first symptoms do not appear until after the disease has spread beyond the ovary (Figure 21). Only too often there is evidence of widespread dissemination throughout the abdominal cavity.

Ovarian cancer tends to spread by implantation within the abdominal cavity, although spread via the lymph or the bloodstream to bones, lungs and lymph nodes may occur. One of the most obvious results of multiple deposits settling in the peritoneal cavity is an outpouring of fluid into the cavity, a condition known as *ascites*. This adds to the discomfort of distension associated with ovarian cancer. This tendency to form fluid may involve the pleural cavity around the lungs as well as the abdominal cavity, a complication sometimes called Meig's syndrome.

Treatment

The treatment of ovarian cancer is removal of the affected ovary by surgical operation. The disease is very commonly bilateral so that, even if the other ovary appears normal, in many instances it is wise to remove both this and the uterus as well, particularly in a post-menopausal patient. Surgeons often remove the uterus as part of the radical operation for ovarian cancer because, with endometrioid cancer,

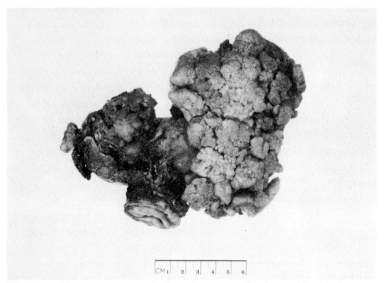

Figure 21 Trans-serous spread of ovarian cancer. Surface exfoliation from a serous papillary carcinoma

there is a definite incidence of unsuspected malignancy in the uterus. Nevertheless, hysterectomy is probably superfluous once there is widespread intra-abdominal disease, though removal of the main tumour mass is regarded as helpful.

If the disease is confined to the pelvis, then radiotherapy may be used. Although most of the patients thus treated will eventually die of the disease, useful palliation may be achieved. When the disease has spread throughout the abdominal cavity, radiotherapy has little to offer. In the past such patients have almost all died within a year.

Since the early 1960's an additional form of therapy has been available, namely the use of cytotoxic anti-cancer drugs (such as cyclophosphamide). In about 40 per cent of patients useful palliation may be achieved with cytotoxic therapy and in a small number, perhaps some 15 per cent, prolonged and unexpected survival may be achieved. These drugs are, however, dangerous and even carry a mortality in their own right. Indeed, not only are they dangerous, but in many instances they are extremely unpleasant. Their side-effects include nausea, vomiting, diarrhoea, ulceration of the mouth and loss of hair. This latter is a very important and distressing symptom to a patient, particularly if she has not been warned about it in advance. It is, however, possible to obtain a wig under the National Health Service and it is prudent to make arrangements for this before the loss of hair begins.

As cytotoxic agents are general tissue poisons rather than specific anti-cancer agents, the brunt of cytotoxic therapy is taken by the actively dividing body tissues such as the bone marrow. Indeed, one of the most dangerous complications of such therapy is depression of the bone marrow (the site of both red and white blood cell formation). One of the first signs of toxicity is a reduction in red cells (anaemia) which may go on to involve all the blood cells (aplastic anaemia). If the white cells are reduced to a very low level (agranulocytosis) or removed altogether, then the body's ability to resist infection is grossly impaired. Under these circumstances, it is infection which may be responsible for the mortality of therapy. Gross reduction in blood platelets (thrombo-cytopenia) may be responsible for a marked tendency to bleeding, with spontaneous bruising and haemorrhage at many different sites.

Cancer of the ovary remains a depressing disease and a nurse in a gynaecological ward should be aware of the gloomy outlook and also of the complications of treatment. An important part of her duties will be to provide support for the patient and her relatives in the terminal phase.

Disorders of the oviducts

By contrast with the ovary, cancer of the oviduct is extremely rare. On the other hand, inflammation is common. Acute inflammation is known as *salpingitis* and is usually bilateral. Salpingitis may present as an acute abdomen and is very similar in many ways to appendicitis. There are, however, one or two important differences. The oviduct is open at both ends and receives a blood supply from two sources, from the uterine and ovarian arteries. Therefore, in contrast to the appendix, gangrene and perforation are very rare. Acute salpingitis may be non-specific, that is to say, associated with no specific infecting organism, but occasionally inflammation is directly due to gonorrhoea. It is important to recognize that this may be the first manifestation of gonorrhoea in the female.

Acute salpingitis may subside with treatment and leave very little in the way of permanent damage to the tubes. On the other hand, it is a condition that may well progress to chronic inflammation and, in this case, permanent damage to function is very likely. One of the first effects of salpingitis of this nature is that the fimbriated ends of the tubes become matted together and the end thus becomes occluded. The result is that the tube becomes a closed organ similar to the appendix and it may distend (Figure 22) and fill up with pus (*pyosalpinx*). Such enlargement of the tube is maximal in the free or ampullary portion. It is frequently adherent to the back of the broad ligament and in the pouch of Douglas produces what is traditionally referred to as a 'retort-shaped' swelling.

Pyosalpinx is undoubtedly associated with destruction and damage to the delicate lining of the tube so, even if it is successfully treated, the chances of having a normally functioning tube in the aftermath are extremely slight. If such a swelling does settle down and the infection is cured, there may remain a blocked and distended tube filled, not with pus, but with a clear fluid (*hydrosalpinx*, see Figure 22). Both these conditions are associated with infertility since the occluded tube is unable to pass the oöcyte down to the uterus.

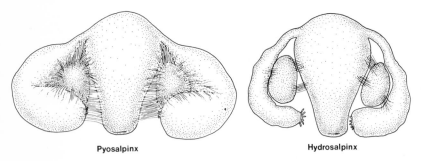

Pyosalpinx   **Hydrosalpinx**

Figure 22 Pyosalpinx and hydrosalpinx

Inflammation may not always matt together the fimbriated ends of the tubes. Chronically diseased and thickened tubes may exist without obstruction to the lumen. The general term *chronic pelvic inflammatory disease* is often used and rarely the ovary and the tube may fuse together to form an abscess cavity (*tubovarian abscess*). Most chronic cases do not have a specific cause, though occasionally the cause may be tuberculosis.

Genital tuberculosis is similarly associated with infertility, and may also involve tuberculous inflammation of the endometrium. Endometrium is shed every month and the detection of endometrial tuberculosis therefore requires that a sample of endometrium be collected just before a period is due. Such a premenstrual endometrial biopsy is obtained by curettage (see p. 40). Evidence of tuberculosis may be found by histological examination or by bacteriological culture. In rare cases, tuberculosis may involve the cervix or, more seriously, may produce different forms of peritoneal inflammation, including the production of ascites (see p. 61) with miliary (widely scattered) intra-peritoneal spread. In more advanced cases the menstrual cycle is disturbed and, in particular, periods may be reported by patients to be scanty or absent.

Chronic pelvic inflammatory disease is common in tropical countries, and in Europe there is an increased incidence of this condition in immigrant patients. Besides infertility, the complaints may be of heavy periods, pain on intercourse and abdominal pain at other times. If the disease is mild, the patient's only complaint may be infertility and, therefore, the elimination of tuberculosis will be one of the important and early steps in the investigation and treatment of infertility.

Infertility

It goes without saying that it takes two to make a pregnancy and that the male partner must be examined in the assessment of any infertile marriage. One of the first investigations of an infertile couple must be to examine the male ejaculate for the presence of live germ cells (spermatozoa). If this test is found to be abnormal in any way, then it is unreasonable to persist with the investigation of the woman, as the tests are sometimes painful and carry a slight risk. The seminal examination may be made on fluid retrieved from the woman some hours after intercourse (post-coital test), and this confirms the presence of live spermatozoa in the mucus of the cervical canal.

Investigations

Besides the examination of the endometrium, the investigation of infertility consists of studies of the patency of the oviducts. The simplest method is injection of carbon dioxide through the cervix. If the tubes are patent (open), gas will bubble into the peritoneal cavity, where it may be detected by an observer listening through a stetho-scope placed on the abdomen. This test, known as *tubal insufflation* (Figure 23), performed on the unanaesthetized patient, is comparatively crude. It is possible to use a radio-opaque dye instead of gas, a process known as *hysterosalpingography*. The progress of the dye may be observed on an X-ray screen as it flows through the tubes into the

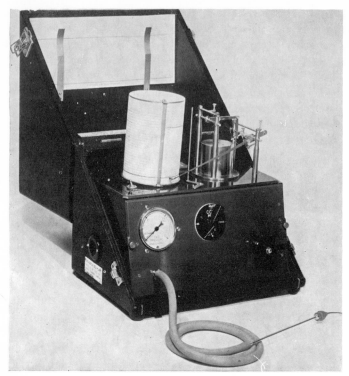

Figure 23 Equipment for tubal insufflation – kymograph machine

abdomen. If the tubes are free from disease, the dye will readily pass to the distal end where a free spill into the peritoneal cavity may be seen. X-ray pictures are referred to as *salpingograms* (Figure 24).

One of the modern ways of investigating the oviducts is by *laparoscopy*, which allows direct inspection of the ovaries and tubes and, if blue dye is injected through the cervix at the same time, the exact site of blockage may be visualized. The technique of laparoscopy is described in Chapter 6 (p. 97).

Treatment

If these investigations reveal blockages in the tubes, operations can be performed to by-pass them. When the distal ends of the tubes are blocked, the operation, known as *salpingostomy*, involves making a fresh opening in the tube. If the block is in the portion of the tube which

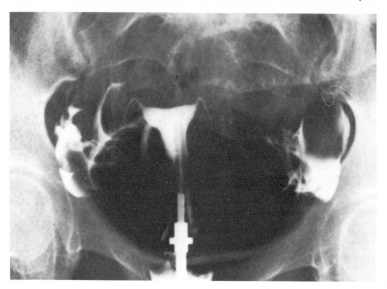

Figure 24 Salpingogram

runs through the uterine wall (and such a block may follow uterine infection after either an abortion or even normal childbirth), it is possible to divide the tube, which may be healthy beyond the block, and re-implant it into the uterus. In this case the operation is known as *uterotubal re-implantation*, or anastomosis.

Although diseases of the tube account for most of the mechanical causes of infertility, a small number of cases are associated with failure of the ovary to produce oöcytes at the appropriate time, a condition known as *anovulatory infertility*. The treatment of this very small group of patients has received publicity out of all proportion to the incidence of the complaint. Such patients may be treated by drugs which are specifically designed to promote ovulation. The most important of these drugs is known as clomiphene, but more rarely a special preparation of follicle stimulating hormone may be used. The unbalanced use of these drugs is responsible, on very rare occasions, for multiple ovulations, resulting in multiple pregnancies and the rare conception of quintuplets.

Besides the complication of unwelcome multiple pregnancy, the use of these preparations in infertility has other risks. Under certain circumstances the treatment is responsible for the production of ovarian cysts which may be subject to all the recognized hazards of ovarian cysts (torsion, rupture or internal haemorrhage), and indeed these cysts may be associated with tremendous outpouring of fluid from the serous membranes, so much so that a state of shock may be induced.

These serious complications of treatment imply that the management of infertility forms an important part of specialist gynaecological practice. The anxiety of the patients and their relatives may require considerable tact and skill in handling by the nurses who have to deal with them. It must also be remembered that within a marriage strains may have been induced by the feeling that one or other partner was to blame.

Sometimes a couple will decide to accept artificial insemination with semen from a donor. Occasionally the husband's own semen may be used, usually when there is some mechanical bar to copulation.

Summary of nursing points

The oviducts are sometimes the site of infection and the nurse must acquaint herself with the features – such as lower abdominal or acute abdomen pain. Occasionally infected tubes may rupture and give rise to peritonitis. Large ovarian cysts may embarrass respiration, or they may obstruct the ureters, rectum and the venous return from legs.

In cancer of the ovary serious effusions and abdominal swelling are common. The care and support of patients undergoing anti-cancer drug therapy are now important parts of a nurse's work and inevitably this involves terminal care of the dying patient and her relatives.

The nursing of infertility patients requires tactful handling of both marital partners and avoidance of chance remarks which could apportion blame.

Chapter 5

Disorders of the vagina and vulva

The *vagina* is a fibro-muscular tube some 8 cm long lying below the uterus and providing it with a communication to the exterior between the lips (labia) of the *vulva*. The axis of the vagina in the standing position is at approximately 45 degrees to the horizontal and is thus nearly 90 degrees to the axis of the uterus. This angulation is of some importance, as it is a factor in preventing displacement of the uterus (see p. 100).

Anatomical relationships of the vagina

The relationship of the vagina to neighbouring organs (Figure 25) is of considerable importance. The upper end of the vagina is called the *vault* and the cervix (see p. 16) projects into this, where on palpation it feels rather like the tip of a nose. The four arches round the vault caused by the projection of the cervix are each called a *fornix*. The posterior fornix is related to the peritoneal cavity, the pouch of Douglas. Below the peritoneal reflection the posterior vaginal wall is closely related to the rectum down to the point where the latter becomes the anal canal, when it bends backwards and away from the vagina. The intervening space is filled by a wedge of fibro-muscular tissue called the *perineal body*.

In front, there is no relationship with the peritoneum as the bladder completely covers the anterior fornix. The bladder is an intimate relation of the anterior vaginal wall in its upper two-thirds and the urethra in the lower one-third.

Structure of the vagina

The vaginal tube, including the cervix, is lined by an epithelium essentially the same as skin without the horny layer. Although the main vaginal tube is derived from the paramesonephric (Müllerian) ducts, the epithelium grows up from below (the sinovaginal bulb), and this type of squamous epithelium is not represented in other structures of paramesonephric origin.

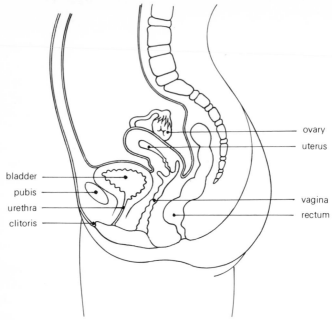

Figure 25 Relationship of vagina to surrounding organs

The vaginal lining is relatively resistant to infection. It has to withstand the trauma of intercourse and later of childbirth, for which the vagina has to be capable of considerable distension. The front and back walls are normally in apposition (close together) but, in a state of shock, the tone in the vaginal walls may be lost so that quite a large volume of blood can be accumulated within. One of the reasons why the vagina is resistant to infection is that it is more acid than many other parts of the body. Really the only micro-organism that thrives in this environment is Döederlëin's lactobacillus, which is not a pathogen and is partly responsible for the acidity. If anything occurs to alter this acidity, the vagina may become susceptible to infestation with other organisms.

Vaginal discharge

One of the commonest complaints that may take a woman to her doctor is vaginal discharge. Discharge may be a nuisance by its mere presence, or it may, in addition, be offensive and cause soreness or irritation.

Rarely the cause may lie above the vagina. Pus may be discharged into the vagina from within the uterus (*pyometra*), usually associated with old age, or from a pelvic abscess through the posterior fornix. Occasionally a small fistula may present as vaginal discharge, the true nature of the complaint not being apparent.

More usually the cause of vaginal discharge lies within the cervix or vagina. The cervix is often responsible for vaginal discharge, as the normal endocervical epithelium is high columnar and mucus-secreting in character. The junction between this epithelium and that of the vaginal portion, known as the squamo-columnar junction, may vary in situation, and sometimes this junction is well out on to the vaginal portion, so that the tip of the cervix appears bright red and weeping. This is a condition known as a *simple erosion* (Figure 26). It is most

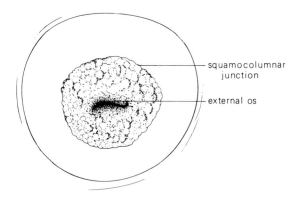

squamocolumnar
junction

external os

Figure 26 Cervical erosion. The glistening papillary area is covered with glandular epithelium

common in sexually active women, but may be present in virgins. The condition may well be hormone-dependent, because there is a tendency for it to appear in women on the contraceptive pill. A simple erosion is responsible for an excessive, clear, mucoid discharge which, however, may dry brown on the underwear. The treatment is destruction of this excessive columnar epithelium by cautery or freezing in the hope that it will be replaced by scar tissue and squamous epithelium. This often requires administration of a general anaesthetic.

The columnar-cell-lined glands of the endocervix, and in particular those which spread on to the ectocervix (the outer cervix) as an erosion, very easily become infected, in which case the character of the discharge changes from mucus to that of mucopus, and the condition of *chronic cervicitis* develops. There is then an ebb and flow of the 'tide' of the squamo–columnar junction and the squamous epithelium may grow back over the mouths of exposed glands, which then get retained as cysts filled with mucopus, often known as *Nabothian follicles.*

This is the stage known as chronic cervicitis and, besides being responsible for chronic discharge, is believed by many to be responsible for chronic pelvic pain, dyspareunia (pain on intercourse, see p. 88) and occasionally recurrent urinary tract infections. The treatment is much more radical than that of a simple erosion and diathermy destruction (destruction by heat, usually electrically induced) or surgical excision of the whole area is indicated. This will often involve a stay in hospital for around ten days, the procedure being known as *conization.*

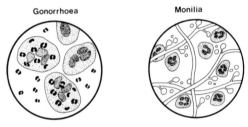

Figure 27 Causes of vaginal discharge

Even the entirely normal cervix may be the seat of an acute inflammation (*acute cervicitis*) when this is inflamed and angry and exuding pus. Acute cervicitis is highly suspicious of an infection with the gonococcus, the organism responsible for gonorrhoea (Figure 27). It is important for a nurse to realize that vaginal discharge may be the only symptom of gonorrhoea in the female and, indeed, discharge is such a common symptom that the woman may be totally unaware that there is anything amiss. The gonococcus tends to affect only columnar epithelium and so the endocervix is acutely inflamed, together the urethra and paraurethral glands and sometimes the orifices of Bartholin's glands, which lie towards the posterior part of the vestibule.

Gonorrhoea, therefore, needs to be excluded from the diagnosis of any patient who has purulent vaginal discharge, and the doctor who is taking swabs in such an examination will need to take these swabs from the cervix and not just the traditional high vaginal swab. He will also wish to take swabs from the urethra and from the anal canal. These swabs must not be put straight back into the tube from which they came, but must be put into a small pot of transport medium, which will prevent the swab from drying out and prevent the rather delicate gonococcus from being killed. The transport medium is known as Stuart's transport medium, and often special swabs which have been previously treated with charcoal are used (Figure 28), but this is not essential.

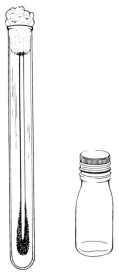

Figure 28 Charcoal swabs and Stuart's transport medium

Cancer of the cervix (see p. 43) may be responsible for vaginal discharge, not only in its own right, but by causing pyometra above. The discharge tends to be blood-stained, and blood-stained discharge should always be regarded as of the same significance as intermenstrual bleeding.

Other vaginal disorders

Inflammation of the vagina itself

The vagina is lined with stratified squamous epithelium and is remarkably resistant to bacterial infection. There are, however, two main causes of vaginal inflammation (*colpitis*), both due to a nonbacterial infecting agent. The first is the yeast *Candida albicans*. This produces a raw-beef appearance and a sore and irritating vagina with white plaques and a curd-like discharge. Irritation is a very prominent feature with this yeast infection, which is also known as *monilia*. Although yeasts are allied to fungi, they are not amenable to treatment with systemic fungicides, and the only treatments of avail are local mycostatic agents, which are applied in the form of pessaries or creams. Occasionally an old-fashioned remedy, painting with Gentian violet, may still be used. Certain conditions predispose to monilial infections, namely diabetes mellitus, pregnancy, the contraceptive pill, antibiotic therapy and debilitating illness, together with immunosuppressive or cytotoxic therapy (see p. 62).

The other common vaginal infection is due to a protozoan organism (a single-celled animal) known as the *Trichomonas vaginalis* (Figure 29).

Trichomonas

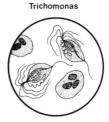

Figure 29 *Trichomonas vaginalis*

This is a motile organism the same size as a white blood cell. It is responsible for producing an acute inflammation of the vagina, but may on occasions be found in the vagina with little or no general evidence of its presence. In an acute infestation the vagina is reddened with punctate (pin-point) haemorrhages and filled with a greenish, slightly frothy pus.

The diagnosis is best made by microscopic examination in the clinic of a drop of pus stirred up with one drop of normal saline on a glass slide under a cover slip. A nurse who is assisting in a gynaecological clinic will frequently be asked to make up a 'wet slide' preparation for the doctor to look at. It is important not to flood the slide with too much saline. The trichomonas is spotted by the movements it makes amongst the clumps of white cells which constitute the pus.

This disorder is responsible for soreness and irritation, but it never causes serious systemic disease. It is believed to be a sexually transmitted disease and is readily treated by a course of tablets (metronidazole) which are usually given to both partners in a sexual union.

There are a few other rare causes of vaginal infections of which the *Herpes virus* is one that is receiving increasing recognition.

Cancer of the vagina

This is extremely rare, and treatment from the nursing point of view does not differ greatly from that of extensive carcinoma of the cervix (see p. 44). This cancer may be secondary to a primary cancer elsewhere, usually in the uterus, sometimes choriocarcinoma (see p. 118).

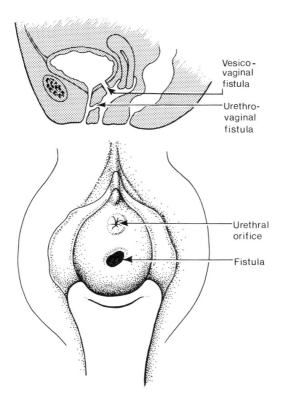

Figure 30 Vesico-vaginal fistula.

Vaginal fistulae

Although not common in the Western world, vaginal fistulae form one of the most important aspects of gynaecological practice in developing countries. Many of these fistulae are the end result of neglected and infected obstructed labour and usually (Figure 30) involve the bladder (*vesico-vaginal fistula*). The sufferers are frequently young girls who, as a result of this harrowing experience in their first pregnancy, are left as permanent social outcasts, smelling of the urine that permanently drips from them. As well as psychological distress, the patients commonly suffer from malnutrition and, because of infection, much of the vagina and part of the uterus will have sloughed away. A rectal fistula may complete the misery. The skill and care of the nursing staff are vitally important in the treatment of this condition.

Preoperative nursing care

The vulval skin is likely to be eroded and excoriated (raw) due to the urine and must be healed before any repair is attempted, so a prolonged period of preoperative nursing is essential. If there is an associated rectal fistula, it is usual for faecal diversion to be performed first in the form of a transverse colostomy. The patient is then nursed face-down on a Stryker bed or Bradford frame (Figure 31) to allow the urine to drip free of the vulva and the excoriated perineal area straight into a bedpan beneath the hole in the bed. Various barrier creams and lotions will be used on the excoriated area to promote healing. Attention must be paid to diet and the correction of parasite infestations, and physiotherapy provided for the contractures (foot

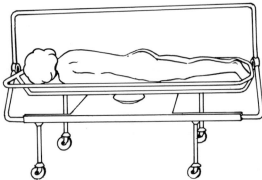

Figure 31 Stryker bed or Bradford frame. The urine drips into a receptacle under the bed without excoriating the vulva

drop) which may have resulted from nerve damage during the obstructed labour.

The operation

Most vesico-vaginal fistulae are repaired by a vaginal approach (Figure 32), though a large relaxing (Schuchardt) incision may be required, which can be quite painful afterwards. High fistulae may occasionally be repaired by an abdominal approach. Owing to the amount of scar tissue that has to be divided, there may be considerable loss of blood during the operation, so shock and haemorrhage may result.

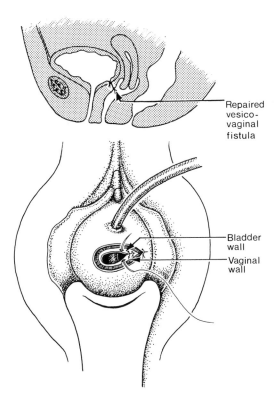

Repaired vesico-vaginal fistula

Bladder wall

Vaginal wall

Figure 32 Correction of vesico-vaginal fistula by separating the bladder and vagina and sewing them up as separate layers

Postoperative nursing care

After the operation, the patient will have an in-dwelling catheter inserted. This is not the Foley catheter used in other types of gynaecological surgery, for the balloon of such a catheter would lie on and press against the precarious suture line where the fistula has been closed. Instead, a large straight whistle-tip catheter is used; this may have a sleeve on the outside which may have been sewn to the vulval lips. This is the only way of ensuring that the catheter stays in exactly the same position, although it causes considerable discomfort.

It is the constant maintenance of satisfactory catheter drainage that is the keystone to success in fistula surgery, and this is where the attention of the nursing staff is so important. As the surgery has been carried out on the bladder itself, the urine will be contaminated with blood, and clots and sediment will form within the bladder. If these block the catheter, tension will build up in the bladder and the stitchline will soon be disrupted. Once a leak has occurred, it will rarely close spontaneously.

The nursing routine is therefore to measure carefully and record the hourly output of urine. Any major difference in output from one hour to the next must be reported immediately to the doctor as, at this stage, it may be possible to unblock the catheter and re-establish drainage.

Drainage is usually maintained for two weeks, but the patient's problems will often continue owing to the damage caused to the bladder-neck-closing mechanism during the obstructed labour. Moreover, the bladder, having drained through a hole for so long, will be small and fibrotic with a very small capacity. So, to maintain continence, the patient must be offered a bedpan hourly after the catheter has been removed. Gradually the time between bedpans will be increased, allowing the bladder capacity to increase.

Occasionally, owing to massive urethral destruction, full urethral control may never be regained, and urinary diversion must be considered. In developing countries, this may pose considerable problems as abdominal diversion of urine into a bag is usually unacceptable and the patients may have to accept uretero-colic anastomosis (with its attendant risk of kidney infection). Such patients pass a mixture of urine and faeces per rectum.

Treatment of rectal fistulae follows similar lines and, if a colostomy was performed in advance, closure of this will be the last item in the long series of surgical procedures these unfortunate patients must undergo.

Gynatresia

This is the term which is given to absence of the vagina or to stricture formation which renders it too narrow for sexual intercourse. *Congenital gynatresia* may be the result of a gross hormonal or chromosomal defect; the vagina is represented only by a dimple in the perineum between the labia minora (see p. 80). Sometimes this defect occurs without other genetic disturbances and is an isolated failure of development of the paramesonephric ducts from which the female genital tract develops (see p. 17). The construction of an artificial vagina is therefore a problem for a plastic surgeon. This may be achieved by opening up the space between the urethra and the anal canal and inserting a split skin graft. Nowadays a more simple method is used, devising a tube of skin from the vulva and enclosing this over the area where a vagina would have been.

Acquired gynatresia is a secondary phenomenon. It may be related to the insertion of noxious chemical substances into the vagina by amateur abortionists, resulting in severe scarring and stricture formation, or the sloughing of the vagina after infected and obstructed labour. Occasionally, however, such strictures may be related to over-enthusiastic surgery for prolapse (see p. 108) or may be the result of infections. If a normal uterus is present above such a stricture, the menstrual discharge may be retained and the resultant distension of the uterus with blood is known as *haematometra*. If the stricture involves only part of the vagina, the upper vagina may be similarly involved, in

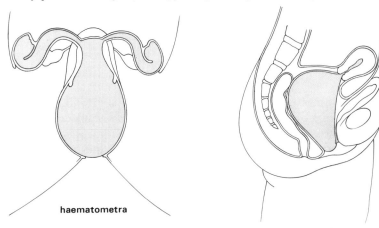

haematometra

haematocolpos

Figure 33 Gynatresia

which case the term used is *haematocolpos* (Figure 33). This is most commonly seen in the congenital form with an imperforate or intact hymen (see p. 19).

Anatomy of the vulva

The main lips of the vulva (the *labia majora*) are the most superficial structures (Figure 34). Between them lies a small hooded structure (*the clitoris*), which is the female phallus and is the equivalent of the male penis. Like the penis, the clitoris is capable of erection and is responsible for much of the sensation experienced during sexual intercourse. The two flaps of skin which form a hood over the clitoris

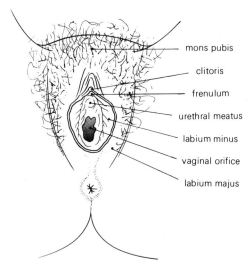

mons pubis

clitoris

frenulum

urethral meatus

labium minus

vaginal orifice

labium majus

Figure 34 Anatomy of the vulva

fade out posteriorly. These are the small lips (the *labia minora*) and their size varies considerably, often undergoing atrophy in older women. Anteriorly, each of the labia minora splits into two components which surround the clitoris – the *prepuce* in front and the *frenulum* behind. On either side of the labia minora are flattened, roughened areas of the skin which are the counterpart of the male scrotum.

At the lower end of the vagina there is a 'lobby' sometimes referred to as the *vestibule* which lies between the labia. The vagina opens into the vestibule, as does the urethra, which lies anteriorly and discharges on to a small eminence, the *external urethral meatus*. There are two small pits on either side known as the *paraurethral fossae*. The detailed anatomy of this area is of considerable importance to the nurse, who may be required to pass a catheter into the urethra. She must always remember the existence of the paraurethral fossae since attempts to pass a catheter into either of these will inevitably contaminate the catheter and will not succeed in producing a flow of urine. It so happens that the para-urethral fossae are sometimes easier to spot than the urethral meatus itself. The clitoris forms a useful landmark above and should be identified.

Posteriorly there is a small pit which lies between the *hymen* and the fold of skin (the *fourchette*) between the lips of the vulva. This pit is called the *navicular fossa*. The hymen itself is a flap of skin, often half-moon shaped, which partially occludes the lower end of the vagina. This usually has one or more holes in the middle sufficiently large to transmit a small finger. The hymen must be stretched at the first act of intercourse, a process known as defloration commonly associated with some bleeding. It is finally disrupted with the birth of the first baby. The small tags which are left are referred to as *carunculae myrtiformes*.

The pubic region

Above the vulva and clitoris there is a region of fat overlying the pubic bone which bears hair in both sexes. It is known as the mons veneris after Venus, the mythical Goddess of Love. The distribution of pubic hair is different in the female, and a flat bar of hair is usual instead of a triangle of hair extending to the umbilicus (navel). The development of hair and of the other structures mentioned occurs at puberty with the other secondary sexual characteristics. Occasionally such development does not occur and this may be an outward sign of a major genetic abnormality, which will normally also involve a failure to menstruate.

Abnormalities

At birth, inspection of the genitalia constitutes the accepted method of distinguishing sex. Occasionally the external genitalia are ambiguous and there is no immediate answer to the question 'What sex is the baby?' Enlargement of the clitoris and partial fusion of the labia may be superficially indistinguishable from penile hypospadias (in which the urethral orifice opens on the underside of the penis) and undescended testes. Besides genetic abnormalities, there is an important metabolic cause (*adrenogenital syndrome*) for this condition of intersex: an enzyme failure in the adrenal gland causes certain substances similar to male hormones to be produced instead of the normal cortisol. The baby may therefore become seriously ill through lack of cortisol.

Either at puberty or later, the vulva may exhibit changes which make it more closely resemble the male genitalia. This process is known as virilization and the most obvious features are an increase in the amount and distribution of hair and an increase in the size of the clitoris (*clitoromegaly*), usually accompanied by a failure of menstruation (*secondary amenorrhoea*). When virilization is suspected, careful endocrine studies are required, and inappropriate levels of male hormone may occasionally be found, usually produced by a masculinizing tumour of the ovary.

Disease of the vulva

Most of the pathology of the vulva is inflammatory in origin. Acute vulvitis is, however, relatively uncommon. In children, acute vulvo-vaginitis may be due to gonorrhoea picked up in the parents' bed.

Venereal disease

In adults with gonorrhoea, inflammation is largely confined to the urethral mucosa, the para-urethral glands and two glands within the labia minora. These glands (Bartholin's glands) discharge within the vestibule in a postero-lateral position and are responsible for the secretions during sexual activity. Inflammatory discharge in these positions should arouse suspicion of gonorrhoea and special swabs (usually charcoal swabs) will be required as for inflammation of the cervix. The nurse will likewise eventually be asked to put these swabs into Stuart's transport medium for carriage to the laboratory.

It is important to realize that venereal disease in women can be symptomless in its early stages. The primary lesion of syphilis is the chancre (a small painless lump which marks the point of entry of the infection), and this is likely to be internal and invisible. Later there may be enlargement of lymph glands with more general manifestations such as a rash and snail-track ulcers in the mouth. One of the lesions of secondary syphilis is the venereal wart. These warts (*condylomata lata*) become flat and ugly and are teeming with the infecting spirochaetes of syphilis. The standard Wasserman blood test for syphilis does not become positive until after the primary infection.

Vulval warts

Venereal warts should be distinguished from the more common viral warts (*condylomata acuminata*), which have a fronded papillary appearance. These may be found in the vagina and anal canal, as well as on the vulva (Figure 35). They may, however, be associated with other genital infections, and infection with the protozoan *Trichomonas vaginalis* (see p. 74) is common. Condylomata acuminata are treated by podophyllin paint or cautery under anaesthetic. The associated infection must also be treated.

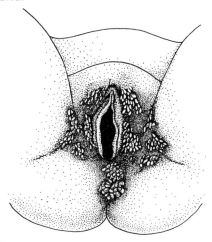

Figure 35 Vulval warts

Bartholin's glands

The ducts of Bartholin's glands may become blocked and form cysts in the gland. These require drainage by the operation of marsupialization, which involves the creation of a fresh aperture for the dilated duct within the vulva. Sometimes the blocked ducts become infected, in which case an abscess develops – a very painful condition. This requires efficient drainage using a similar technique.

Elephantiasis of the vulva

Bilateral swelling of the vulva is rare in temperate climates and is usually due to lymphoedema secondary to chronic lymphatic obstruction. A quiescent tuberculous infection of the lymph nodes may be responsible.

Chronic vulvitis

Chronic vulvitis may occur on its own without evidence of vaginal infection. Symptoms may be either soreness or irritation and, of the two, irritation is perhaps the most prominent. Any of the conditions mentioned (p. 70) as producing vaginal discharge may produce secondary irritation of the vulva, but some of them may only affect the vulva. For example monilial infection of the vulva may well be missed if only a vaginal swab is taken in search for the diagnosis.

Certain general diseases, particularly skin diseases, may present with skin changes and irritation of the vulva, and these need to be considered. By far the most important is diabetes mellitus which may present with a vulvitis not due to monilia, although the two may often co-exist, and the nurse can be instrumental in making the diagnosis by making sure that the urine of all patients presenting with vulval irritation is tested for sugar.

When the skin of the vulva is chronically inflamed, the cells of the area may be so disturbed that they become *premalignant*. A general term for the characteristic appearance under these circumstances is *leukoplakia* (Figure 36). This is a term which is also used to describe white plaques occurring on the lips or tongue, and which likewise may have a premalignant connotation. In the mouth there is a strong association with syphilis, which is not the case with leukoplakia on the vulva. There tends, however, to be some confusion in the terms because not all conditions which produce white skin changes on the vulva are leukoplakia; the term is therefore best used for those changes which indicate an unrest of epithelial cells which could lead to malignancy.

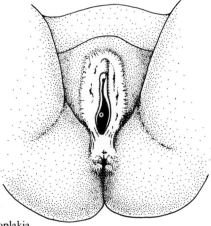

Figure 36 Leukoplakia

The treatment for vulval skin conditions is usually local application of special ointments, but very occasionally the local area of skin requires to be excised. This is not a major operation, although it may give rise to a certain amount of postoperative pain. Certain specific infections and infestations can produce vulval irritation in addition to those mentioned and the crab louse (*Pediculosis pubis*) and scabies (Figure 37) and tinea cruris (a fungal infection) all have to be considered in some instances.

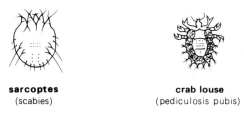

sarcoptes
(scabies)

crab louse
(pediculosis pubis)

Figure 37 Parasites of the vulva

In tropical countries, certain granulomatous conditions can affect the vulva and perineum. These may occasionally be seen in immigrant patients in Europe. The best known of these is *Lymphopathia venereum*, a sexually transmitted disease characterized by fibrosis and tissue destruction. The vulva, including the terminal urethra, is largely destroyed and recto-vaginal fistula and rectal stricture may occur. The Frei test is used for diagnosis and depends on a skin reaction to an injection.

Vulval cancer

Cancer may affect the skin of the vulva, this is occasionally secondary, but usually primary. Skin cancer is normally regarded as radiosensitive, but in the particular situation of the vulva, radiotherapy is not really suitable because the necrosis produced by radiotherapy produces very unpleasant sloughing and soreness of the area concerned.

Treatment

The surgery of vulval cancer involves one of the biggest procedures with which a nurse will deal in the care of gynaecological patients. The operation (*radical vulvectomy*) involves a very wide local excision of vulval cancer (Figure 38) going deep into the buttock areas on either side of the vagina, a dissection of the groins and the lymph nodes

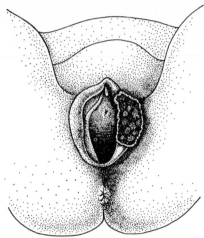

Figure 38 Radical vulvectomy. A small carcinoma can be seen on the right labium minus

around the main vessels to the leg, and often division of the inguinal (groin) ligaments with dissection of lymph nodes within the pelvic cavity. Frequently the terminal urethra requires to be removed as well. There is thus a very large raw area which cannot usually be closed completely. This area almost invariably becomes infected and breaks down so that the period of postoperative nursing in hospital may extend to several months.

Postoperative nursing care

These patients are best nursed under a cradle so that the stitch lines may be kept as dry as possible, but a considerable amount of fluid may seep from the exposed raw areas. The patients will require very considerable psychological support because they will have little conception of how mutilating the operation may seem. A nurse must be prepared for this and must not allow herself to be shocked when she first inspects the operation wound when the patient returns from the operating theatre. Many of the reactions which a patient can show to the disfigurement of mastectomy (removal of the breast) will occur in patients who undergo radical vulvectomy, but the reaction tends to be more delayed. Sometimes further operations and skin grafting are necessary to close the raw areas. On the credit side is the fact that the results of surgical treatment tend to be better than they would be for cancer in many other parts of the body.

Summary of nursing points

The main conditions affecting the vagina and vulva are discharge, carcinoma, fistulae and inflammation.

The nurse must be able to assist the doctor as required when vaginal smears and swabs are required.

Where infection is of venereal origin, the nurse must ensure that everything is done to prevent its spread. She must be particularly careful when carrying out procedures of an intimate nature, such as vulval swabbing and toilet; gloves must be worn.

Where surgery is indicated for vulval cancer, the nurse must be aware of the radical nature of the operation and its subsequent debilitating effects, and she must do everything possible to reassure the patient by way of support and counselling.

In the care of patients after repair of fistulae, the supervision of urinary catheter drainage can be crucial to the success of the operation.

Chapter 6

Painful conditions of the female genitalia

Pain in the pelvic or lower abdominal region due to conditions of the uterus, ovaries or oviducts is a symptom which may bring a patient to seek medical advice. More particularly, this complaint of pain may be related to various functions of the genital tract, particularly intercourse and menstruation.

Pain on intercourse

This is called *dyspareunia* and is in general referred to in two main categories. *Superficial* or *friction dyspareunia* is pain or discomfort on penetration by the male and is related to conditions of the vulva and vagina which were considered in Chapter 5. The uppermost part of the vagina behind the cervix is, however, a direct relation of the peritoneal cavity and conditions which are responsible for tenderness located in this part of the peritoneal cavity will be responsible for *deep* or *collision dyspareunia*. This may be distinguished as a deep pelvic pain felt at the limit of the intromittent thrust of intercourse and is a pain which may well persist for some hours afterwards. Normally the pouch of Douglas is empty apart from the empty rectum. A common cause of deep dyspareunia is a full loop of large bowel in this position (Figure 39), so that ordinary constipation ranks high amongst the causes for this complaint.

Retroversion

The uterus itself may be displaced backwards into the pouch of Douglas, a position known as a *retroversion*. Under these circumstances the two ovaries hang down behind, right up against the posterior vaginal fornix and are thus exposed in the same manner to mechanical disturbance. Dyspareunia is really the only symptom which may be attributed to such retroversion and does constitute an acceptable indication for its correction. Mobile retroversion may be corrected by the insertion of a plastic S-shaped ring, called a Hodge pessary (Figure

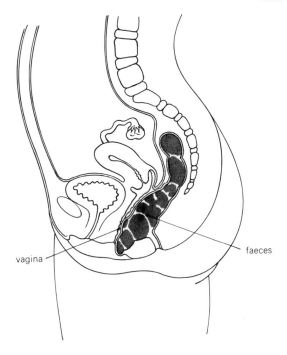

Figure 39 How constipation can cause dyspareunia

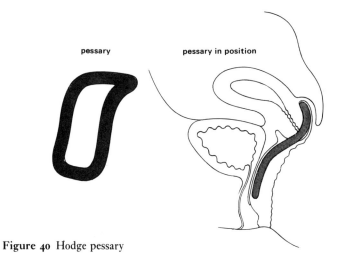

Figure 40 Hodge pessary

40), which will hold the uterus anteverted. If this is successful in relieving symptoms, then many would accept this as an indication for the operation of *ventrisuspension*, which is done through a laparotomy incision and consists of surgical manoeuvres to fix the uterus in an anteverted position, usually by shortening or plicating the round ligaments.

Fixed retroversion

Sometimes the uterus cannot be displaced forwards because of inflammatory adhesions and under these circumstances the insertion of a Hodge pessary would do no good. The commonest cause of such inflammatory adhesions is chronic salpingitis (as described in Ch. 4), but any adhesions after abdominal surgery, particularly in which there has been a leakage of blood, may result in a fixed adherent retroversion. It is therefore quite common gynaecological practice to antevert the uterus at the conclusion of any operation in which this is at all likely.

Endometriosis

In a Caucasian population, another very common cause of a fixed painful retroversion responsible for deep dyspareunia is the condition known as *endometriosis*. This has been mentioned briefly in connection with the cysts of the ovaries (see p. 59), but it is a condition which is not confined to the ovaries. In a European community it is an extremely common disorder, about which the general public is singularly ill-informed. It is exceptional to find a lay person who has ever even heard of the diagnosis of endometriosis or, having heard of it, has the least idea of what it is all about.

Pelvic endometriosis is a condition in which islands of endometrium, consisting both of glands and of the surrounding stroma, are to be found in situations outside the cavity of the uterus (Figure 41). The presence of tissue like this in areas which are not normally occupied by such tissue is reminiscent of malignant disease, but endometriosis has no other features comparable to cancer and is indeed believed not to be a form of cancer. In exceptionally rare instances it may undergo cancerous change, as may endometrium in the normal site.

Endometrium in the uterus is highly dependent for its structure upon the influence of hormones secreted by the ovaries. However, the deepest layer (the basal layer) does not respond in the same way. When endometrium is formed in these so-called ectopic sites, it tends mostly

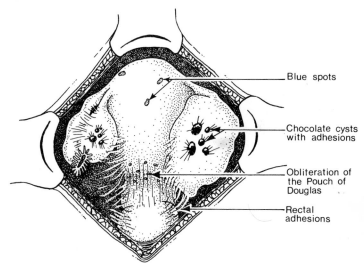

Blue spots

Chocolate cysts
with adhesions

Obliteration of
the Pouch of
Douglas

Rectal
adhesions

Figure 41 Endometriosis

to be of the same type as basal endometrium and, therefore, to show little response to the changing patterns of hormones.

Nevertheless, in any site where there is anything more than a tiny clump of endometrium, the hormone-dependent pattern of the more superficial layers may be seen, and this may include a tendency to bleed at the time of menstruation. In a closed area, of course, this must lead to the loculation of small amounts of blood, which eventually become inspissated (thickened) and altered. Such material appears dark blue when viewed from outside through the wall of a cyst but, when exposed to the light of day, is a deep chocolate colour. The occurrence of large chocolate-filled cysts in the ovary is one of the most prominent features of pelvic endometriosis, but small scarred areas with little blue-domed chocolate cysts within them are characteristic of endometriosis in other sites.

There are a variety of explanations for this strange condition, none of which entirely accounts for all its manifestations. It is well recognized that during menstruation blood from within the uterus may drip back through the oviducts into the pelvis. It is also known that this blood may well contain viable endometrial cells which can be cultivated in appropriate tissue culture media. It is further recognized that the surface of the peritoneal cavity is an appropriate area on which such exfoliated endometrial cells may implant, and this theory of 'retrograde spill' would account for the maximum incidence of endometrial deposits being in the ovary and on the underlying uterosacral ligaments. The theory of implantation is the only one which will account for the occurrence of endometriosis in operation scars, particularly in the scars of abdominal operations when the cavity of the uterus has been opened. The most prominent cause for postoperative scar endometriosis is hysterotomy for termination of pregnancy. This is much more common than in the scars following Caesarean section, for it is believed that by the time pregnancy has reached term the endometrium (then called decidua), is effete and much less likely to implant.

Besides being found in the pouch of Douglas and the ovaries, endometriosis may occur on the peritoneal surface anywhere in the pelvis, such as the vault of the bladder, the round ligaments, the front of the rectum, the sigmoid colon, the appendix and even the terminal ileum (since any structure which may hang down into the pelvis can be affected by endometriosis). It does, however, very occasionally develop in sites outside the peritoneal cavity and, in some of these, it may be difficult to implicate the theory of direct spill. It is known to appear in the lungs, occasionally in the pleura and has been recorded in the axilla and in muscles of the arm. Blood or lymph-borne spread is likely to have occurred in such instances.

The rival view to the spill or spread theory depends upon the fact that the female genital tract develops as the paramesonephric duct from inclusions from the primitive peritoneal cavity and subsequently the coelomic (peritoneal) epithelium is converted into endometrium. This rival theory presupposes that other areas of coelomic epithelium are capable of undergoing the same sort of transformation into ectopic endometrium.

Clinical features

The most prominent clinical feature is pain, and dyspareunia may be one of the obvious varieties. Physical signs which suggest endometriosis are the finding of a fixed, painful retroversion with bilateral appendage swelling and tender nodules in the pouch of Douglas. These nodules may sometimes be felt more readily on rectal examination. There is often an associated complaint of infertility – or perhaps it is that patients who defer having children until the age of 30 or so may be more prone to endometriosis. One of the more remarkable features of this disorder is that the severity of the symptoms may bear very little relation to the extent of the disease. Very localized disease may be responsible for persistent complaint, and some patients with extensive disease deny, even in retrospect, that they have any relevant symptoms.

Treatment

In the first instance, this must be surgical as this is the way the diagnosis is made. Ovarian chocolate cysts may be enucleated and the ovary re-constituted, and the fixed painful retroversion may be corrected by the operation of ventrisuspension. Other areas of endometriosis may be excised or treated with diathermy. In the past, extensive endometriosis was always treated by bilateral oöphorectomy and the disease can always be controlled by the production of a surgical menopause, though nowadays this is considered unnecessarily drastic. In the older age group of patients, for whom conservation is no longer indicated, total hysterectomy with removal of the most diseased ovarian tissue is a fairly standard procedure, but even in these patients it is not uncommon to leave a small amount of apparently normal ovary. In the event of further symptoms they can always be treated at this stage by an X-ray menopause.

Hormone treatment

One of the features of endometriosis is a tendency for the condition to regress if the patient becomes pregnant. As it happens, many of these patients are infertile either involuntarily or by social convention. An attempt has therefore been made to mimic the hormonal conditions of pregnancy by treating the patient with high doses of synthetic gestogens producing a pseudo-pregnancy (not to be confused with pseudo-cyesis, when a patient is deluded into thinking she is pregnant when she is not). Pseudo-pregnancy involves the complete suppression of menstruation by increased doses of a gestogen which are necessary to prevent breakthrough bleeding. This treatment has proved to be only of limited value.

The role of the nurse

Nurses are particularly likely to be involved in explanations to patients about this disease, because patients very rarely understand clearly what is told to them on the first occasion and, when they are told about a disease of which they have never heard, they are very likely to get a mistaken impression. Moreover, some of the features of this disease, as has been pointed out, resemble those of cancer. The misapprehension in this instance may be particularly unfortunate. It is especially important, therefore, for nurses on gynaecological wards to be familiar with this condition and be prepared to discuss it with their patients in an intelligent fashion.

Acute abdominal pain

Gynaecological conditions can be responsible for the development of acute or subacute abdominal pain, which may or may not present as a surgical emergency. A nurse may, therefore, encounter the causative conditions either in the gynaecological ward or quite frequently in general surgical wards.

Severe local pain

Any organ which may undergo torsion (twisting) is liable to become infarcted and its blood supply become interfered with, and this may be

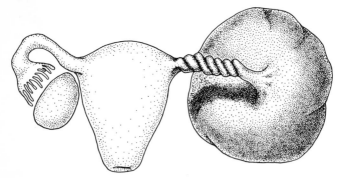

Figure 42 Torsion of the ovary

responsible for very severe local pain. Any swelling of an ovary which causes it to reach a size big enough to have sufficient twisting movement about its pedicle may make it liable to undergo an acute torsion (Figure 42). Such a swelling must be above a certain critical size and yet not so big that it is impacted within the pelvis. On the other hand, if it lies free above the uterus then it can reach a bigger size and still be able to undergo torsion. It is very rare for extremely large ovarian cysts to twist in this fashion. There is often a history of minor attacks preceding the one which has produced a really acute pain. Occasionally cysts may undergo internal haemorrhage from other causes, perhaps associated with malignant change, or even comparatively minor trauma may cause rupture of such a cyst. Very rarely other pelvic organs may undergo torsion and these include the uterus itself, fibroids on small pedicles, cysts of the oviducts, and cysts of adjacent structures.

Diffuse pain and peritonitis

Acute inflammation of the oviduct starts as a local pain, but may well be associated with a spreading peritoneal inflammation so that peritonitis is produced. If a pyosalpinx (see p. 64) ruptures, then there is a diffuse spreading of pus throughout the peritoneal cavity and the patient is very ill. The presence of an inflammatory mass and peritonitis may be extremely difficult to distinguish from a perforated pericolic abscess in diverticular disease or an appendix abscess. The rupture of an ovarian cyst, particularly a chocolate cyst due to endometriosis, may present with the features of general peritoneal irritation without the history of premonitory local warning pain. Perhaps the most important cause of abdominal pain, both of the diffuse variety and of the localized variety is ectopic pregnancy, which will be dealt with in Chapter 8 (p. 115). The pain in this instance is due to an acute or subacute discharge of blood into the peritoneal cavity (*haemoperitoneum*). The same phenomenon, less acute, may be produced by rupture of a small physiological ovarian cyst, a condition sometimes known as *ovarian apoplexy*.

Chronic abdominal pain

In youngish women this is most likely to be associated with pelvic endometriosis or chronic salpingitis (pelvic inflammatory disease) but, in the postmenopausal patient endometriosis is exceptionally rare as a cause for pain and the possibility of malignant ovarian disease needs to be considered. The manifestations of ovarian cancer (see p. 60) are entirely non-specific. Chronic pain in premenopausal women is usually only ascribed to gynaecological conditions if there is a relationship to menstruation.

Dysmenorrhoea

Painful periods are known as *dysmenorrhoea* and the condition is so common that it is often made light of, though it can be a very crippling burden that some women have to endure.

Spasmodic or primary dysmenorrhoea

This is the colicky pain associated with the onset of flow, typically present in young women. It may be associated with vaso motor disturbances, such as fainting, sweating and even nausea and vomiting. A nursing sister in any organization where young women are employed will be called upon to render First Aid on innumerable occasions to sufferers from this condition. The pain very rarely precedes the onset of menstruation by more than a few hours and classically lasts a day or two; rarely, it is worse on the second day. The pain characteristically only occurs with the contractions of the uterus which has been primed by progesterone and, in other words, does not occur if ovulation has not preceded the episode of vaginal bleeding.

The first few cycles which produce vaginal bleeding in a young girl at puberty are quite commonly anovular and therefore pain-free, so such a girl may well give a history that her first few periods were painless. In the same way, suppression of ovulation by hormone therapy, such as the contraceptive pill, may well bring about relief from spasmodic dysmenorrhoea. This type of pain may also improve once regular sexual activity has begun, for reasons which are obscure, but in particular it is unusual after a pregnancy. In some way dilatation of the cervix makes it easier for the blood to be discharged and the same colicky contractions are not set up. This type of dysmenorrhoea in the past was treated by dilatation of the cervix, but this manoeuvre is now less popular as it may lead to damage to the cervix which could predispose to subsequent abortion. Both pain and tension before a period is due may possibly be related to unbalanced production of prolactin and local production of prostaglandins.

Membranous dysmenorrhoea

This type of dysmenorrhoea, ascribed to the passage of a uterine endometrial caste, is regarded as very rare, but pain with menstruation associated with the passage of clots ('clot colic') is very common and this is a feature of heavy periods which are also painful.

Secondary or congestive dysmenorrhoea

This term is applied to the onset of painful periods later in life, usually in a woman in which periods have not been painful for a number of years. The condition is characterized by a crescendo of pain preceding menstruation and which is often, but not always, relieved by the onset of the flow. This type of painful menstruation is usually secondary to some organic pelvic pathology, in contrast to primary dysmenorrhoea which occurs in an anatomically normal uterus. The conditions responsible for secondary dysmenorrhoea are most usually pelvic endometriosis or pelvic inflammatory disease. In particular, endometriosis which is confined to the body of the uterus, and to which the term *adenomyosis* is sometimes applied, is a likely cause.

Where dilatation of the cervix may sometimes be of value for spasmodic dysmenorrhoea and may improve the situation where menorrhagia is giving rise to clot colic, it is not anticipated that it would provide any relief for secondary dysmenorrhoea. In this instance the underlying cause needs to be treated and occasionally this may require hysterectomy. If, however, conservative surgery is being carried out for a condition such as endometriosis, it may on rare occasions be justifiable to divide the nerve pathways which transmit the impulses from the lower part of the uterus. These lie in association with the sympathetic nerves in the hollow of the sacrum and are, therefore, called the presacral nerve by surgeons. The operation for their division is known as a *presacral neurectomy*.

Laparoscopy

In the investigation of lower abdominal pain endoscopy and X-ray studies of the urinary tract and bowel form an important part of the investigation. The genital tract may be felt more easily by examination under anaesthesia (EUA), but even this is a relatively inaccurate method. Exploratory laparotomy is occasionally necessary without a firm diagnosis and a lesser measure available is peritoneal endoscopy, now known by the rather inappropriate name of *laparoscopy*. In this procedure, a special needle with a spring-loaded safety cover to the point (to protect the bowel from injury) is passed through the abdominal wall and some four litres of carbon dioxide are instilled into the peritoneum (Figure 43). It is advisable to use a pressure manometer because it can be serious if the end of the needle is in the wrong place, such as in the mesentery. Once a pneumoperitoneum has been induced, X-rays may be taken which show the ovaries (*pelvic-pneumography* or *gynaecography*) but more usually an endoscope with a large trocar is inserted which allows inspection of the pelvic viscera.

It is as well for nurses to be aware of the fact that this is by no means the minor procedure it seems and is certainly not comparable to cystoscopy or sigmoidoscopy. Intraperitoneal bleeding may occur just as after any laparotomy with the production of shock or many of the late sequelae of abdominal surgery. Full postoperative observations are required and such patients are rarely let out of hospital earlier than 48 hours from operation. Furthermore, the anaesthetic is not the simplest as the abdominal distension may embarrass respiration and, if the gas leaks under pressure into the tissues, surgical emphysema will be

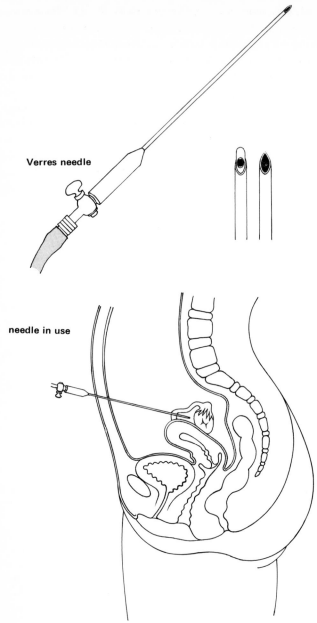

Verres needle

needle in use

Figure 43 Laparoscopy. Induction of Pneumoperitoneum

produced, sometimes reaching the mediastinum, and serious circulatory difficulty may arise. Nevertheless, laparoscopy is increasing in popularity and in its place is a very useful investigation; it has an expanding role as a means of carrying out sterilization by diathermy coagulation of the oviducts.

Summary of nursing points

The painful condition of endometriosis is common. As the patient is unlikely to have heard of this condition, the nurse must be able to explain it to her, and must be aware of the accompanying clinical features of infertility dyspareunia and dysmenorrhoea. The nurse should appreciate the potential hazards of laparoscopy and the early features of possible complications.

Chapter 7   Prolapse and displacements

The term *prolapse* implies dropping or protrusion of an organ. Although vaginal prolapse and uterine prolapse are separate entities, they are so commonly associated that it is convenient to consider them together. The term prolapse is not confined to descriptions of the genital tract and, in general surgical wards, the nurse may be familiar with prolapse of the rectum – a condition in which the rectal mucous membrane is turned inside out and protrudes from the anus. Rarely the same phenomenon may occur to the female urethra, particularly in young children, as prolapse of the urethral mucosa. When applied to the female genital tract, the term does not imply the same unrolling phenomenon. It means rather a dropping or sliding down (Figure 44).

Inversion

In this condition, the uterus itself turns inside out. *Inversion* is

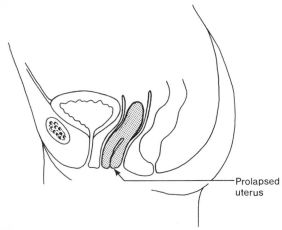

Prolapsed
uterus

Figure 44 Prolapse of the uterus

scarcely seen in the non-pregnant state, and a chronic inversion can only arise as a result of the neglected inversion of a pregnant uterus, with the possible exception of the protrusion through the cervix of a submucous fibroid (see p. 42) attached to the fundus of the uterus.

Uterine prolapse

Prolapse of the uterus implies descent of the intact uterus down the length of the vagina with eventual extrusion outside the vulva. To understand what is involved and the mechanisms of treatment it is necessary to refer again to the basic anatomy. The uterus sits like an inverted pear above the hollow tube which is the vagina. There is little obvious suspension from above, and it would be logical to suppose that the force of gravity, aided by straining and raising of intra-abdominal pressure, would tend to push the uterus down the vagina, like a piston pressed from above. One should perhaps therefore consider why *all* women do not suffer from such prolapse of the uterus. One reason is that the uterus does not normally lie in the axis of the vagina, but is angled forwards over the vault of the bladder in the position known as *anteversion* (Figure 45). In addition, the anterior and posterior vaginal walls normally lie flat together so there is only a potential space down which the uterus could be expelled by a bearing-down effort. After

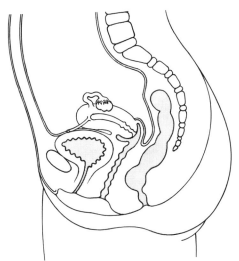

Figure 45 How anteversion normally prevents prolapse. The axis of the uterus is nearly at right angles to that of the vagina.

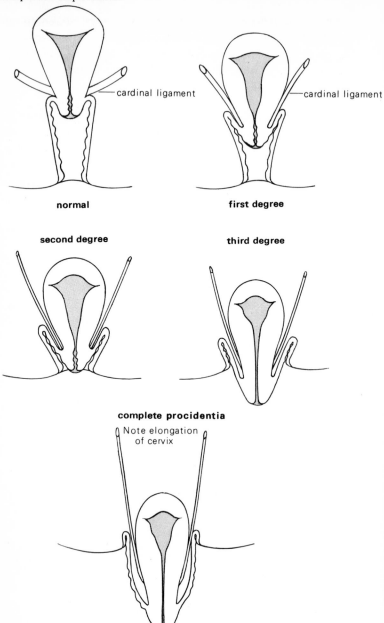

Figure 46 Prolapse of the uterus

childbirth this space may be opened up and in some women, of course, the position of anteversion is not maintained.

The first prerequisite, therefore, for uterine prolapse is that the uterus should point directly down to the vagina. It will then be in a position to be propelled down the vagina by forces acting from above. It is normally retained within the pelvis by two ligamentous structures which spread fan-wise from the cervix to the lateral walls of the pelvis, beneath the flimsy broad ligaments. These structures are known as the *transverse cervical* or '*cardinal*' ligaments. From their appearance from above, it is easy to understand why they are sometimes colloquially referred to as the 'butterfly' ligaments. If these become stretched like the 'guy' ropes of a tent, they allow the uterus to descend on straining.

Uterine prolapse is classified into four degrees (Figure 46):

$1°$ descent within the vagina
$2°$ descent so that the cervix reached the introitus
$3°$ descent with the cervix protruding outside
$4°$ the vagina is turned inside out (also called procidentia).

Vaginal prolapse

By contrast, vaginal prolapse is a true protrusion or hernia of the vaginal wall into its lumen and, in due course, this also may extend through the vulva to the outside. Like any hernia, vaginal prolapse must contain an underlying organ, and thus the organs which lie immediately adjacent to the vagina, both front and back, form the contents of a vaginal wall prolapse.

Anterior vaginal prolapse

The most obvious prolapse of the anterior wall is known as *cystocele* (Figure 47); this is a protrusion of the upper two-thirds of the anterior vaginal wall into the lumen, and contains the bladder.

The lowest one-third of the anterior vaginal wall is related to the urethra. This is more firmly held to the back of the arch of the symphysis by the triangular ligament and urethral suspensory ligaments and, therefore, a major protrusion in this area is unusual. However, stretching and dislocation of these ligaments allows a corresponding swinging forwards of the urethra and tends to roll the lowest part of the vagina into the introitus. This phenomenon, seen best on straining, is sometimes called 'cartwheeling' of the urethra, and may also be called *urethrocele* (Figure 47).

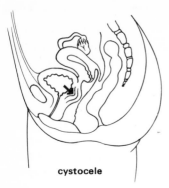 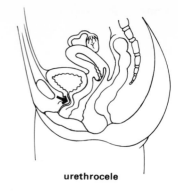

cystocele   urethrocele

Figure 47 Anterior vaginal prolapse

Posterior vaginal prolapse

The posterior vaginal wall is related in its upper quarter to the pouch of Douglas, and any protrusion of this particular region must contain a true peritoneal sac; this is referred to as an *enterocele*, or hernia of the pouch of Douglas. The middle segment of the posterior wall is directly related to the extra-peritoneal rectum, and a bulge in this region is known as *rectocele* (Figure 48). The lowest quarter of the posterior vaginal wall is related to the fibro-muscular body known as the perineal body. Although this is not the content of a prolapse, partial division of the perineal body in childbirth makes possible the lower protrusion of a rectocele. Therefore deficiency of the perineal body is commonly associated with the problems of posterior vaginal wall prolapse.

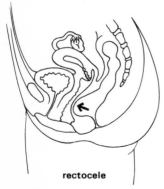 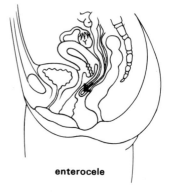

rectocele   enterocele

Figure 48 Posterior vaginal prolapse

Symptoms of prolapse

Descent of the uterus into the vagina will produce dragging on the cardinal ligaments and utero-sacral ligaments and may produce a vague sacral backache. But, in general, backache is a symptom which arises from conditions of the back and it is wise not to ascribe backache too readily to minor degrees of gynaecological prolapse. In second-degree prolapse the uterus descends right to the introitus so that the patient has a feeling of a 'lump' being present, and indeed may have a sensation of wishing to bear down, reminiscent of the process of giving birth to a baby. The same reflexes may be involved as in the involuntary expulsive efforts of the second stage of labour, but of course to a lesser degree. If the uterus comes right outside the vulva, the patient will complain of a palpable or visible lump.

Vaginal wall prolapse may produce symptoms related to the adjacent viscera. The only symptom of rectocele may be the presence of the lump, possibly with some difficulty in evacuating the rectum. Straining at stool may merely balloon the rectocele without achieving evacuation and occasionally the patient will say that she has to press back the lump before she can manage to pass a stool. The bladder, however, is a more

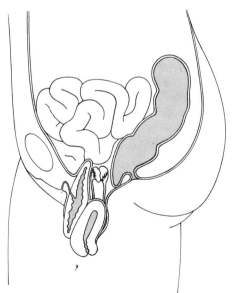

Figure 49 How major prolapse can prevent micturition

sensitive organ and symptoms of cystocele may arise from mechanical irritation of the bladder base and produce frequency of micturition. This sensation is usually relieved at night when the prolapse is reduced. Any patient who complains of nocturnal frequency should, therefore, be suspected of having some other intrinsic lesion of the bladder besides cystocele, and the same may well be said for the symptom of urgency of micturition.

With major degrees of uterine prolapse there may be actual kinking of the urethra and inability to pass urine (Figure 49). Such a patient may rarely present with acute retention of urine or even chronic retention with overflow. It is very important to realize that, in major degrees of prolapse, the urinary tract obstruction may be at the uretero–vesical junction, producing back pressure in the ureters and hydronephrosis (distension of the kidney by retained urine) and even, on occasions, uraemia (excess urea – and other waste products – in the blood). This is the only complication of genital prolapse which is a threat to health or life; prolapse is otherwise a disorder of social inconvenience and discomfort.

The dislocation of the supports of the urethra may give rise to the particularly distressing social phenomenon known as *stress incontinence* of urine.

Stress incontinence

Stress incontinence is the involuntary leakage of small amounts of urine when intra-abdominal pressure is raised, such as may occur in coughing, laughing, lifting or straining. It may vary from a very minor symptom, producing momentary embarrassment requiring the occasional changing of underwear, to such wetness occurring at the least movement that the patient requires to wear a pad and becomes sore and smells of urine.

About two-thirds of patients who have stress incontinence have some degree of anterior vaginal wall prolapse of the cystocele variety. It is convenient, therefore, that procedures designed to repair the cystocele will usually restore the anatomy of the urethro–vesical junction sufficiently to allow a woman to regain control over micturition in moments of stress. Probably the explanation is that minor degrees of utero–vaginal prolapse prevent the upper urethra being protected and squeezed by the act of raising intra-abdominal pressure and thus urine is forced into the upper urethra, which is normally empty. Even this does not always make a woman wet, since the small external voluntary sphincter muscle may be able to act as a second line of defence. If, however, this has been damaged in the process of childbirth, a small amount of urine will be allowed to leak. Correction of minor degrees of utero–vaginal prolapse may restore the upper urethra to its normal intra-abdominal position. The pressure differential within the urethra is thus maintained during raising of intra-abdominal pressure and thus continence is preserved.

About one-third of patients with stress incontinence do not have significant utero–vaginal prolapse and the treatment under these conditions is much more difficult. sometimes a minor vaginal operation of the repair type may be successful but, on other occasions, more involved abdominal procedures involving suspension of the bladder neck region to the anterior abdominal wall or back of the symphysis pubis may be necessary.

Treatment of prolapse

Genital prolapse is essentially a mechanical problem, and the treatment must be mechanistic and, therefore, surgical. In a few patients where surgery is inappropriate, the prolapse may be retained by an apparatus worn within the vagina known as a *ring pessary* (Figure 50). This expands the vaginal vault above the gap in the levator ani muscles and acts as a platform on which the prolapsing uterus may sit. It also

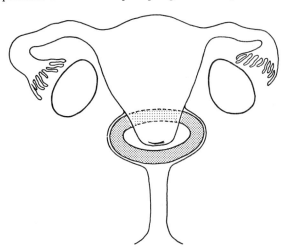

Figure 50 Ring pessary in position

distends the anterior and posterior vaginal walls, preventing them from prolapsing so easily.

Vaginal pessaries may be used as a therapeutic test to determine whether symptoms ascribed to a minor prolapse can in fact be relieved by its correction. They may also be used to provide temporary relief when prolapse occurs after childbirth while the supports of the uterus and the enlarged vagina are shrinking back to the normal non-pregnant state. Such rings need changing at intervals, usually three or four times a year. In the past, old-fashioned rubber rings were used and have occasionally been forgotten by patients. Such rings can set up very nasty ulceration, and this has, on rare occasions, turned malignant.

The operations

As uterine and vaginal prolapse almost always go together, the operations are designed to cope with both features. The standard principles of hernia repair are applied to vaginal wall prolapses, namely excision of redundant tissue, building up a firm layer of tissue to support the gap which is left, and resuturing the overlying skin. These are known as *colporrhaphy* operations, either anterior or posterior. The posterior colporrhaphy or *repair* is usually associated with a reconstruction of the perineal body, known as perineorrhaphy.

Uterine prolapse is treated by one of two procedures. Firstly, a vaginal hysterectomy and repair may be carried out (Figure 51). This involves removal of the entire uterus, but not the ovaries or oviducts, through the vagina. The stump of the round ligaments and tubes are then sutured to the vaginal vault to act as supports for this structure. In patients with prolapse, extensive anterior and posterior colporrhaphies are also necessary. Vaginal hysterectomy may also be performed when there is only minimal prolapse; but some other reason for hysterectomy, such as abnormal periods, is usually present in this case.

The alternative operation is known as the *Manchester repair* (Figure 52). This is an ingenious procedure designed to counteract the various features which have led to uterine prolapse. The underlying principles are the exposure of the overstretched cardinal ligaments from below and their effective shortening by suturing together in front of the cervix. This, at the same time as elevating the uterus, pushes the cervix backwards and restores the position of anteversion, which prevents subsequent prolapse. The situation is made complete by amputation of the elongated cervix which is part of the pathology of uterine prolapse.

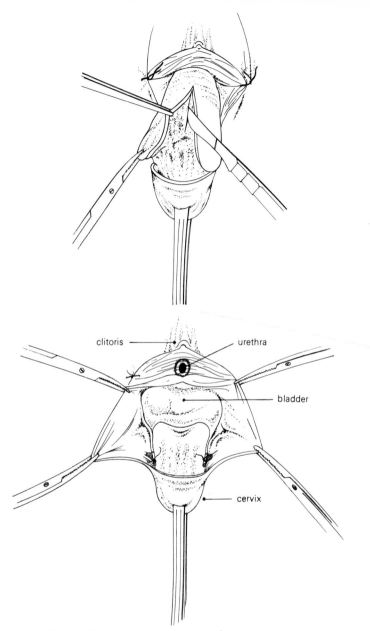

Figure 51 Repair of prolapse; the vagina is inside-out

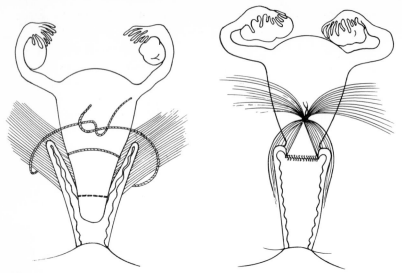

Figure 52 Manchester repair. Amputation of cervix and plication of cardinal ligaments

Nursing care and complications

Preoperative care

The same investigations and preparations are required as for abdominal hysterectomy (see p. 48), except that any patient with a major degree of uterine prolapse should also have a blood urea estimation as well, in case there has been urinary tract obstruction. If the cervix has been protruded for any length of time, it may be severely ulcerated and under these circumstances the doctor may prescribe rest in hospital with local treatment to prepare the tissues for operation. The prolapsed uterus has to be retained with a pack soaked in glycerine and paraffin, and treatment with oestrogens is often given as well. In some units, preoperative douching may still be used. The prolapse may be secondary to some other factor which leads to raising of intra-abdominal pressure, such as bronchitis or chronic constipation and straining. Both of these medical conditions may need preoperative preparation, including physiotherapy.

The routine care before a vaginal operation includes a perineal shave (but not an abdominal shave) and bathing using a bactericidal soap.

As with abdominal surgery, the issue of prescribed night sedation and discussion with the patient at the time of getting the consent form signed are the responsibility of the nurse in charge. Normally this latter should occur when the doctor explains the nature of the operation.

Elderly patients may not be worried about sexual function following an operation for prolapse, but to younger women this may be important and, if a nurse suspects that the patient has not declared her true feelings on the subject, it is important that she should speak to the surgeon about this because the detail of each operation can, and should, be tailored to suit a woman's individual needs. There is no doubt that operations for major degrees of prolapse run less risk of recurrence of prolapse if they are carried out so extensively that the vagina is rendered very narrow. This point is important if sexual relations are desired subsequently.

Postoperative care and complications

Postoperative management is very similar to that of an abdominal hysterectomy, except of course, that there is no abdominal wound. The early complications of shock and haemorrhage can well supervene, but it is usual if haemorrhage occurs for there to be overt bleeding from the vagina. This does not always happen, however, and haemorrhage from a pedicle in a vaginal repair can bleed in a retroperitoneal space. This may well produce a large intra-abdominal haematoma with the complications of shock, followed by paralytic ileus and, in the long run, even such remote complications as subphrenic abscess.

The postoperative nursing care of these patients may therefore be summarized as follows:

Immediate:
1. attention to the airway and respiration
2. checking pulse and blood pressure
3. inspection of vulval pad for bleeding
4. attention to catheter drainage
5. pain relief
6. maintenance of intravenous infusion.

After some hours:
1. washing the patient
2. attention to oral hygiene
3. encouragement of oral fluids
4. attention to catheter or vulval toilet and regular abdominal palpation to detect a full bladder or other painful swelling

5. encouragement of deep breathing when appropriate.

Later:

1. mobilization
2. attention to bowels
3. perineal toilet (for which a bidet is ideal)

Most of these patients will have an intra-vaginal pack inserted in the theatre, and this will require removal 24–48 hours after operation. It may be appropriate to give a small dose of postoperative analgesic prior to removal of the pack because, even though it is not likely to cause pain, the patient is liable to be anxious. The only painful part of prolapse operations is the perineal repair. Anterior repair is comparatively painless, but posterior repair can cause considerable bruising, swelling and discomfort around the anus, comparable to stitches after childbirth, or even to the pain associated with a haemorrhoid operation. Complaint of severe pain in the hours after operation should lead to careful inspection of the vulva, because this may be the first sign of the development of a haematoma below the levator-ani muscles which may require evacuation and drainage. Secondary haemorrhage, pelvic abscess and fistula formation can all follow vaginal surgery, just as they can follow any abdominal surgery. The nurse in attendance must therefore be aware of such possibilities if the patient's postoperative course departs from normal. In all gynaecological or pelvic operations, there is an increased hazard of thrombo-embolism and pulmonary embolism and, in the older age group of patients who tend to constitute those most likely to need vaginal operations, this may be a particular problem. Even though such patients may have an in-dwelling catheter, early mobilization is an important part of postoperative nursing.

The in-dwelling catheter is not a feature of every vaginal repair operation, and the practice varies from unit to unit. Many units, however, would regard a period of free drainage with an in-dwelling catheter as preferable to the discomforts of retention and intermittent catheterization, which so often accompany repair done without catheterization. It is comparatively ràre for the urine of a patient with prolapse to be infected before operation, but it is very common afterwards, since the combination of bruising of the bladder and catheterization prove an ideal means for infection. It is, therefore, usual for the doctor to prescribe some urinary antiseptic such as *nitrofuran-toin*, to be taken while the patient has a catheter in place.

The care of the patient trying to re-establish micturition devolves particularly on the nursing staff. Pain and retention at this time can cause considerable distress – to some patients more than the operation itself does. The nurse must observe the frequency and volume of voided urine: increasing frequency with reducing volume implies the development of retention with overflow. It is probably better to put the catheter back for 48 hours than to persevere with running taps and baths and so forth in the face of this situation.

As with abdominal hysterectomy, the patient should be warned about timing and possible difficulty with resumption of married relations following discharge from the hospital and also advised, as for any hernia repair, against lifting or straining for a matter of some months. There is one final procedure which is important after vaginal surgery and that is for the doctor to perform a vaginal examination before discharge from hospital. This serves two purposes, one is to make sure that no form of swab has been left behind within the vagina, and the second is to break down any possible adhesions between the stitch line in the vagina and the opposite vaginal wall. These are soft at this stage but, if left to the postoperative visit, may be quite difficult to break down and can cause bleeding and distress at this time.

Summary of nursing points

The nurse must be aware of the underlying conditions which give rise to prolapse of the uterus and of the vagina. She must also be aware of the main symptoms of prolapse, such as the presence of a lump in the vagina, frequency of micturition, stress incontinence and sometimes backache.

The conservative treatment is diet and physiotherapy to improve the tone of the muscles of the pelvic floor, coupled with the use of pessaries. Surgical treatment consists of the operations of colporrhaphy, Manchester repair and vaginal hysterectomy. The nurse must understand the principles of preoperative preparation, which must include reassurance and allaying any apprehension the patient may have as to the outcome of the operation. After the operation, the nurse must look out for signs of shock and haemorrhage. Most patients will have an intra-vaginal pack *in situ* on return to the ward, and this will require removal in 24–48 hours. Analgesics must be given as prescribed. The nurse must also attend to the in–dwelling catheter if there is one in place and at the appropriate time supervise the re-establishment of spontaneous micturition. The patient must be given breathing and limb exercises, and should be got out of bed as soon as possible.

Chapter 8   Disorders of pregnancy

By tradition, disorders of early pregnancy are considered to be within the scope of gynaecology. Nowadays, however, the distinction is not finely drawn, and midwives recognize the obligation to provide the total care of patients throughout pregnancy. Nevertheless, it is true to say that complications of early pregnancy are dealt with in the gynaecological wards, and a gynaecological nurse must be prepared to cope with the special circumstances of pregnancy.

Abortion

A pregnancy which lasts for six months (28 weeks) or more is said to be *viable* and one which comes to an end within that period of time is said to undergo a *miscarriage* or an *abortion*. There is no difference between these two words. Spontaneous abortion may occur at any time, but most commonly occurs at or around three months. The fetus and the gestation sac, whose formation was discussed in Chapter 2 (p. 27) are discharged from the uterine cavity by a process of dilatation of the cervix and intermittent uterine contractions, a miniature labour exactly equivalent to that which occurs near term for a viable fetus. This process is accompanied by loss of blood. A painless loss of blood from the pregnant uterus is called a *threatened abortion*. The term threatened is used because, in certain instances, the pregnancy can continue without harm until viability. This is because bleeding may occur from parts of the endometrium to which the gestation sac is not yet attached.

If regular uterine contractions accompanied by dilatation of the cervix develop, then the abortion is said to be *inevitable* and it will go on to reach one of several conclusions. If the fetus alone is discharged leaving behind the rest of the gestation sac and miniature placenta, the abortion is said to be *incomplete*. This is always associated with bleeding and usually requires evacuation of the retained products of conception, a surgical operation which needs to be carried out in hospital. If the pregnancy is very early, or conversely more than about four months in duration, then the placenta and membranes or gestation sac may be discharged intact with the fetus and the abortion is said to be *complete*.

Occasionally after a threatened abortion the fetus dies, but there is minimal bleeding and neither the fetus nor gestation sac are discharged. This state of affairs is known as a *missed abortion*.

Septic abortion

In addition, an incomplete abortion may be complicated by infection; this is referred to as a *septic abortion*. A septic abortion is usually, but not always, the result of interference with a pregnancy, whether legal or otherwise (but particularly the latter). A septic abortion may have very serious consequences, producing pelvic peritonitis and septicaemia. The former may be responsible for permanent sterility associated with considerable pain and ill health, and the latter may prove fatal owing to endotoxic shock or acute renal failure.

Unskilled attempts at abortion may produce a serious hazard for reasons other than the introduction of these serious infections. These reasons include perforation of the uterus and adjacent viscera, introduction of gas into the circulation (producing air embolism), and severe haemorrhage.

Ectopic pregnancy

Another important complication of pregnancy arises when implantation (see p. 26) occurs in a site other than in the uterus. This may be in the peritoneal cavity, on the ovary, in the cervix or in the oviduct. The last named is by far the most common site. Ectopic pregnancy is very important because the uterus is the only organ which is correctly adapted to contain an expanding gestation sac. The trophoblast which is formed very early from the products of conception has the property of invasion. This may be contained by the uterine wall but, in other situations, can be very dangerous as it can involve erosion of blood vessels. The problems of ectopic pregnancy, therefore, are really those of internal haemorrhage, which may be acute, subacute or chronic.

Acute or ruptured ectopic pregnancy

In the narrow isthmic portion of the tube there is absolutely no 'give' which will allow expansion of the gestation sac, and a pregnancy in this situation will very rapidly erode through the tubal wall and burst, producing free intraperitoneal haemorrhage. The history may be characteristically catastrophic. About the time a period is due or when the period is a few days overdue, a young woman presents with acute abdominal pain, classically associated with pallor and fainting and often with the additional history of pain referred to the shoulder as a result of irritation of the underside of the diaphragm by blood which has tracked up. A fulminating intraperitoneal rupture of an ectopic pregnancy is a dire emergency. The operative treatment is comparatively simple and very rewarding, but speed is of the essence and such patients are usually admitted straight to the operating theatre without further ado apart from signing a consent form. Rapid transfusion is required and, in difficult circumstances, the blood which is free in the abdomen may be used (auto-transfusion).

Subacute ectopic pregnancy

This is an altogether less urgent business. A pregnancy which arises in the ampullary portion of the tube may well expand this without disruption for some time, even eight to ten weeks from implantation. It will, however, often produce symptoms as a result of bleeding from the end of the tube into the peritoneal cavity. A subacute ectopic pregnancy is often a source of diagnostic confusion, and the pain and bleeding may be confused with a variety of conditions, from varieties of abortion to appendicitis.

Chronic ectopic pregnancy

This is a much slower version of the subacute ectopic pregnancy and the history may go on for many weeks. The presentation may be extremely bizarre. The blood which has been shed slowly from the fimbriated end of the tube into the peritoneal cavity will usually clot around the tube and behind the uterus in the pouch of Douglas. Loops of bowel may well adhere to this clot so that the presentation may be surgical, as intestinal obstruction. Alternatively, the collection of blood within the pouch of Douglas, known as a pelvic haematocoele, may be responsible for pressure on the bladder causing retention of urine, or irritation of the bowel causing diarrhoea, so that the diagnosis may not be suspected for quite some time.

Ectopic pregnancy is well named 'the appendicitis of gynaecology'. The diagnostic problems are, if anything, greater than those of appendicitis.

Diseases of the trophoblast

Vesicular mole

This degenerative disease of placental tissue is sometimes known by the confusing term 'hydatidiform mole'; the term 'hydatidiform' indicates an appearance similar to that of hydatid disease, and the word 'mole' is from the Latin word meaning mass. The term vesicular is preferred, meaning 'a mass of vesicles'.

When a zygote is formed by an act of fertilization it divides to form a mass of cells called the *blastocyst*. At this stage the cells begin to differentiate into those which are going to form the embryo, and those (the trophoblast) which are going to form the accessory tissues. Occasionally the embryo fails to form, and overgrowth of the trophoblast occurs. Normally trophoblast is vascularized by vessels from the fetus but, if the fetus is absent, there will be no blood vessels within the chorionic villi of the trophoblast. In vesicular degeneration

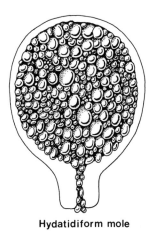

Hydatidiform mole

Figure 53 Vesicular mole

there is, except in the rarest of instances, no fetus and therefore no fetal circulation within these degenerate villi. They swell up and become oedematous, each individual villus varying in size from a pin-head to that of a currant (Figure 53).

In a molar pregnancy, therefore, the uterus contains, instead of a gestation sac with a placenta, a mass of shapeless chorionic villi which are often swollen up in vesicles. The patient is 'pregnant', but she is not expecting a baby. She does, however, suffer from all the symptoms associated with pregnancy because the trophoblast is able to produce chorionic gonadotrophin just as in a normal pregnancy.

The symptoms of pregnancy in this instance are often worse, with sickness being a prominent feature. There is the additional hazard of a complication usually confined to late pregnancy called pre-eclamptic toxaemia. This is characterized by an elevation of blood pressure, oedema and proteinuria. A molar pregnancy will, in due course, abort, but expulsion of the mole may well be incomplete and may be associated with very heavy bleeding. The invasive properties of trophoblast are preserved and sometimes exaggerated so that such a mole may penetrate deeply into the wall of the uterus, occasionally right through it.

Such moles may well break off into the blood stream and be carried to the lungs. Their behaviour there is indistinguishable from that of a malignant tumour and they can just as surely kill the patient by obstruction of her pulmonary circulation. This type of malignant mole is sometimes referred to as *chorio-adenoma destruens*. The diagnosis of vesicular mole is extremely difficult as the clinical distinction between it and an early multiple pregnancy may be almost impossible. All patients with trophoblastic disease will secrete chorionic gonadotrophin in the urine and the so-called pregnancy test will be positive, even though the patient is not expecting a baby, and indeed will be positive even if the urine is diluted many times. The diagnosis of vesicular mole is best made with the diasonograph (ultrasonic B-scan), but the ultrasonic fetal pulse detector can also be useful in early pregnancy in helping to demonstrate a normal pregnancy.

Choriocarcinoma

An even more serious disorder of the trophoblast is a highly malignant cancerous tumour known as *choriocarcinoma* (chorion epithelioma).

This tumour, consisting entirely of trophoblastic cells, shows no tendency to chorionic villus formation and always spreads rapidly. It invades local tissue and metastasizes (spreads) via the blood stream to the lungs and to the lower third of the vagina and vulva. Most cases of choriocarcinoma arise as malignant transformation of a previously benign vesicular mole, but a few cases follow an entirely normal pregnancy and delivery and some follow cases of abortion or even ectopic pregnancy.

There may be considerable time lag (years) between the antecedent pregnancy and the appearance of such a tumour, which may present in a multitude of very strange ways with its metastases. For instance, it may present as a pulmonary embolus, as a lung tumour, as right heart failure or as a cerebral tumour.

Choriocarcinoma is extremely rare in Europe, but relatively common in the Far East and to a lesser extent in West Africa as well. The interest of this tumour lies in its curious origin from products of conception. This implies that it is genetically distinct from the host patient which could be the reason why it is one of the few forms of disseminated cancer for which there is a relatively effective form of treatment even when the disease is quite advanced. Very prolonged remissions may be brought about by chemotherapy, so much so that one can begin to think in terms of cure. Certainly radical surgery no longer has a major place in the treatment of what was hitherto an almost uniformly fatal disease. Today some of the women who have been successfully treated may yet go on to have a subsequent normal pregnancy. It is possible to control the treatment of this disease by monitoring the output of chorionic gonadotrophin (see p. 27) and the quantitative measurement of this hormone reflects the amount of viable tumour tissue remaining. Because of the risk of this complication, all patients who have a vesicular mole should be followed up in this way in order to detect the onset of cancerous change.

Unwanted pregnancy

Another major problem of early pregnancy which concerns gynae-cologists these days is the problem of the unwanted pregnancy and its termination. The law on the termination of pregnancy varies in different lands and is largely influenced by the religious and other customs of the people. In the United Kingdom statutory law now covers the termination of pregnancy. Briefly, it states that it is lawful to terminate a pregnancy before viability when the opinion of two registered medical practitioners is given in advance (on the appropriate green form) that the termination of the pregnancy is not a greater hazard to the mother than continuation of the pregnancy on one of four legally approved grounds. These are:

1. the continuance of the pregnancy would involve risk to the life of the pregnant woman greater than if the pregnancy were terminated

2. the continuance of the pregnancy would involve risk of injury to the physical or mental health of the pregnant woman greater than if the pregnancy were terminated

3. the continuance of the pregnancy would involve risk of injury to the

physical or mental helath of the existing child(ren) of the family of the pregnant woman greater than if the pregnancy were terminated

4. there is substantial risk that if the child were born it would suffer from such physical or mental abnormalities as to be seriously handicapped.

There is, in addition, a statutory obligation upon the operator to notify the termination to the Chief Medical Officer of the Department of Health (on an appropriate buff form) within seven days of carrying out the operation. The operation itself may only be carried out within the National Health Service Hospital or in a place specially approved for the purpose of the Act by the Secretary of State for the Department of Health and Social Security.

Nurses are not involved in the ethical decisions on termination, and a nurse may decline, on conscientious grounds, to participate in the procedure. This, however, does not absolve her from the duty of providing general nursing care and emotional support in the ward to the patients who are undergoing termination. These patients may be in particular need of support rather than veiled or implied criticism.

Termination of pregnancy

Up to three months of pregnancy, the size of the fetus (Figure 54) is such that it may be readily grasped by vaginal instruments and broken up and removed. After three months gestation, this dismemberment process becomes increasingly hazardous with risks of damage to the soft tissues by the bones and of incomplete removal of the pregnancy. Traditionally, pregnancy has been terminated by the operation of dilatation and curettage (see p. 40) up to three months and, after that, by an abdominal operation to open the uterus, evacuate the contents and sew it up. This operation (*hysterotomy*) implies a scar upon the uterus which can be a potential hazard in any future pregnancy and also exposes the mother to all the risks of an abdominal operation. In the state of pregnancy this carries a slightly greater risk of thrombo-embolic complications than would be present at other times from a laparotomy. Three more modern methods are becoming available for termination, and doubtless their popularity will increase.

Suction termination

A vacuum aspirator attached to a hollow tube is inserted into the uterine cavity and the contents may be sucked out with considerably

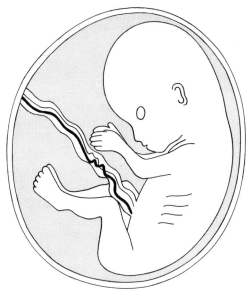

Figure 54 Fully formed fetus at 3 months

less loss of blood than is usual with a formal dilatation and curettage. This may safely be applied to slightly bigger gestation sacs than three months. A modern anaesthetic (*ketamine*) has reduced the amount of bleeding very considerably. During the recovery period the patient may be rather irritable, and nurses should be careful not to disturb her too much. In early cases the operation may be done under local anaesthetic, and this has led to the introduction of an abortion service to out-patients in some centres.

Prostaglandin infusion

Prostaglandins are naturally-occurring substances which act upon smooth muscle, including uterine muscle, and, if injected directly into the uterus, may produce regular uterine contractions even in this early stage of pregnancy. They do, however, produce the unpleasant side-effect of nausea and vomiting, particularly if used by intravenous infusion.

Instillation of abortifacients into the uterus

Hypertonic solutions, either saline or urea, or a combination of urea and prostaglandin, can be instilled into the uterus (Intra-amniotic instillation). This seems to bring about the death of the fetus and is almost always followed by the spontaneous onset of labour and abortion within a matter of a day or two. Sometimes it is necessary to use an infusion of oxytocin to accelerate this. Accidental intravascular instillation of hypertonic saline has grave risks and has even caused the death of the patient. When hypertonic sugar solutions were used, there was a grave risk also of the production of gas gangrene, just as may occur with unskilled attempts at vaginal abortion. Instillation of chemicals (Utus paste via the cervix) has been practised, but as a method of legal termination has virtually disappeared. Prostaglandin may be inserted outside the membranes by a catheter passed through the cervix (extra-amniotic instillation).

The nurse in a gynaecological ward must appreciate that all these patients will undergo a miniature labour before the fetus and placenta are discharged. The professional competence of a midwife is appropriate in this situation, but of course observations on the fetus are not required. The other observations required in labour are important – observations not only of the patient's general condition (including temperature) but of the uterine contractions. The duration, frequency and intensity of these must all be recorded and, in particular, evidence of relaxation between contractions is vital. Tonic contractions can lead to uterine rupture, even during abortions. The progress of the labour may need to be assessed by vaginal examination to determine cervical dilatation. As with any labour, relief of pain and anxiety is paramount. *Analgesia need not and must not be withheld.*

Birth control

The problems of termination are very much bound up with those of unwanted pregnancy and, as with many branches of medicine, prevention is better than cure. The wider problem of population control concerns a variety of interested parties: politicians, agriculturists, demographers and all those concerned with the standard of living and social welfare of mankind. In sophisticated communities unwanted pregnancy is a matter of concern at the family level but, at this level methods of prevention of unwanted pregnancy need to be more reliable than those with a recognized failure rate which may be acceptable as a method of population control. The individual is only concerned with the individual failures, and the fact that 90 out of a 100 other women may have been successfully prevented from having an unwanted pregnancy by the method of contraception used is of little consolation to the woman for whom this method has proved unsuccessful and who is faced with an unwanted pregnancy. Gynaecology is very much concerned, therefore, with developments of methods of birth control and with individual advice to patients on methods which may be suitable.

Sterilization

Apart from removal of the uterus (hysterectomy) there is no absolutely foolproof method of preventing a woman from becoming pregnant if she continues to have sexual intercourse. The most effective methods are those of mechanical sterilization either of the male or of the female. In the male the procedure is known as *vasectomy* and consists of a removal of a short segment of the vas deferens tube which leads from the testis to the ejaculatory ducts. This prevents the spermatozoa (male gametes) reaching the seminal fluid. There is a considerable delay following vasectomy before those spermatozoa which are stored in the seminal vesicles have finally been discharged. During this time other forms of contraception must be used until the semen has been proved to contain no spermatozoa.

In the female the oviducts may either be divided or removed (*salpingectomy*) as the operation of *sterilization*. It is no longer considered sufficient merely to tie a ligature around a loop of tube. The operation may be carried out through a small laparotomy incision and the tubes divided and ligated with proper ligature material. Alternatively the tubes may be divided and coagulated by diathermy through the laparoscope, any bleeding points subsequently being treated by coagulation. Still experimental is sterilization using spring-loaded (Hulka) clips or silastic (Yoon) rings.

Contraception

Reversible methods of prevention of pregnancy involve interference with the process of ovulation, implantation or fertilization (by preventing access of spermatozoa to the upper genital tract).

Ovulation suppression

Contraceptive pills, consisting originally of oestrogens alone and later with a variety of a progestogenic substances added, act by depressing the pituitary production of gonadotrophin and therefore inhibiting the ripening of the Graafian follicles (see p. 15). It was found that continued ingestion of oestrogenic substances produced a small risk of serious thrombo-embolic complications. Although the risk is small, the complications are so serious that the oestrogenic content of contraceptive pills has been reduced. Unfortunately, although this has resulted in no diminution of their efficacy, it has produced an increase in some unwelcome side-effects. Some of the effects of the progestogens in contraceptive pills are disturbing to the patient, particularly loss of libido (interest in sexual activity) and depression. Some patients intensely dislike having their instincts and moods altered in this way for purely social purposes. There is a very low dose continuous gestogen contraceptive pill which acts, it is said, by altering the consistency of the cervical mucus, but as it does not suppress ovulation, it cannot have the same certainty of protection against pregnancy as is present with the modern, more powerful combined pills which contain both an oestrogen and a progestogen.

Intra-uterine contraceptive devices (IUCD or IUD)

A foreign body within the uterus has been used for contraceptive purposes for very many years. Nowadays, these objects are made of inert radio-opaque plastics in a variety of shapes (Figure 55), each of which is alleged by its devisor to be more efficacious than the next. The problems with these devices are extrusion (particularly if unrecognized), colicky pain, uterine haemorrhage, (either intermenstrual or heavy menstrual loss) and, finally, inflammatory disease which also carries a slight risk of ectopic pregnancy.

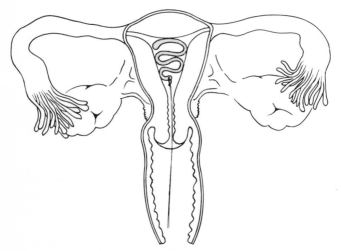

Figure 55 IUCD (Lippés loop) in position

There is also a slight risk of failure even with the device still in the correct place. Some pregnancies can implant and may be successfully established. Nevertheless, this method of contraception has the advantage that, once the device is in place, it requires little or no effort on the part of the woman, merely that she should be alert to the possibility of extrusion. An intelligent woman will learn the art of checking that such à device is in place by feeling for the fine nylon thread which hangs out through the cervix. The failure rate may be further reduced by combination with a spermicidal cream. The latest devices are small enough (Figure 56) to be fitted to a patient who has never been pregnant.

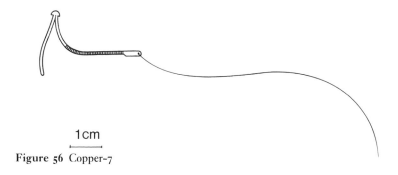

1cm

Figure 56 Copper-7

An important modification to the simple plastic device has been introduced. The Copper 7 (Gravigard) releases a small quantity of copper ions which increase the efficiency of the method. The store of copper is exhausted in about 18 months, so that these devices need changing at more frequent intervals.

Mechanical methods
Obtrusive *diaphragms* may be inserted into the vagina. A less common form is the *cervical cap* (Figure 57), which fits tightly round the vaginal portion of the cervix, but most commonly the vaginal cap lies obliquely across the length of the vagina (Figure 58). This type of device must be fitted carefully by an experienced person and is only really effective if the uterus is anteverted. It must be used in combination with some form of spermicidal cream. It is not really suitable for tropical countries because the rubber material of which the cap is made is liable to perish.

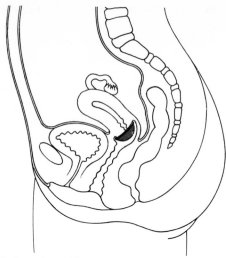

Figure 57 Cervical cap in position

The condom

The male contraceptive is a time-honoured method of prevention which also has the advantage of providing some measure of protection against the acquisition of venereal disease. It is, however, open to the objection of producing some reduction in sensitivity in the male and is likewise subject to technical hazards, such as disruption, pin-hole leakage and even unrolling and coming off during an act of intercourse.

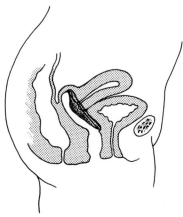

Figure 58 Diaphragm in position

The proponents of family planning point out that the mortality of unwanted pregnancies almost certainly exceeds that of any methods of contraception and, given this fact, there is justification for the use of any of the methods described above. In an individual case, however, there may be factors which weigh for or against any one particular method. For instance, patients who for some reason are particularly at risk from thrombo-embolic disorders would be foolish to use a contraceptive pill for purely social purposes.

The fact remains that in a civilized community every woman should have the right to be free from the tyranny of undesired fertility. It is the duty of all those who practice professionally in the field of gynaecology to provide advice and assistance as required, with the same compassion and understanding that is so necessary in the other aspects of this branch of medical practice.

Summary of nursing points

Most women look forward to a wanted pregnancy and, when something goes wrong which may indicate that the pregnancy will miscarry, the psychological effects on the woman will be considerable. Conversely the tensions from an unwanted pregnancy will likewise be significant, and indeed the patient may be ambivalent in her desire to be rid of it. The nurse must bear this in mind when dealing with such patients; considerable sympathy and tact will be required.

The nurse must be able to recognize abnormalities of pregnancy such as abortion and ectopic pregnancy, which will become evident through loss of blood and pain. Where a patient is admitted to hospital with such conditions, the nurse must see that she has rest, comfort, supervised intake and output and psychological support; at the same time the nurse must make observations of the patient's general condition and watch for signs of shock, haemorrhage or infection.

The nurse must also be aware of other disorders of pregnancy particularly ectopic pregnancy. She must be familiar with the use of contraceptives, and appreciate the vital importance of young women at risk from unwanted pregnancy being properly advised before being exposed to such a risk again. She should be aware that patients should stop taking the contraceptive pill before elective surgery, but that they must be advised to use some other contraceptive method in the interval. She should also note that gastro-intestinal illness such as vomiting or diarrhoea may nullify the contraceptive action of the pill.

Further reading

General
BOOKS

Rosemany Bailey, *Obstetric and Gynaecological Nursing*, Nursing Aid Series, 1969. A good basic guide to the principles of gynaecological and obstetric nursing care.

M. L. Bloom and L. Van Doriger, *Clinical Gynaecology Integration of Structure and Function*, Heinemann, 1972. Clinical and operative application of knowledge of anatomy, physiology, embryology and endocrinology. Written for medical students.

C. W. F. Burnett, revised by Mary Anderson, *A Summary of Gynaecology*, Faber and Faber, 1974. Clear factual information, easy to remember. A useful ward reference book.

G. W. Garland, Joan M. E. Quixley and M. D. Cameron, *Obstetrics and Gynaecology for Nurses*, English University Press, 1973, chapter 2. Particularly helpful list of definition of terms used in gynaecology and obstetrics. Easily assimilated information useful for revision before the State final examination.

Winifred Hector and G. Bourne, *Modern Gynaecology with Obstetrics for Nurses*, Heinemann, 1974. Well illustrated clear account of the nursing skills and understanding required in this speciality.

Chapter 1 Introduction
Anatomy of the genital tract
BOOKS

C. W. F. Burnett, *The Anatomy and Physiology of Obstetrics*, Faber, 1971, chapter 1, pp. 15–37. The Anatomy of the Female Genital Tract. Detailed text illustrated by line drawings.

M. M. Garrey, A. D. T. Govan, C. H. Hodge and R. Callander, *Obstetrics Illustrated*, 2nd edn, Churchill Livingstone, 1975, chapter 3. Obstetrical Anatomy. Entirely diagrammatical representation of the female genital organs. The visual concepts facilitate a clear understanding of structure and position.

B. R. Sweet and I. F. Cape, *Obstetric Care*, Nursing Modules, H.M. & M. Publications, 1976, chapter 2. The Female Reproductive Organs. Complementary to the above.

Development and evolution of the female genital tract
BOOK

J. G. Lewis, *The Endocrine System*, Penguin Library of Nursing, 1973, chapter 1, pp. 164–5. Clear diagrammatic representation of the embryological differentiation of male and female gonads complemented by short text.

ARTICLE

Symposium of General Problems of the Disabled, *Nursing Mirror*, 5 Feb. 1976.

Chapter 2 Ovulation, copulation and menstruation
Ovulation, copulation and implantation
BOOKS

Sir Stanley G. Clayton, D. Fraser and T. L. T. Lewis (Eds.), *Obstetrics by Ten Teachers*, 12th edn, Arnold, 1972, chapter 2, pp. 2–15. Ovulation, menstruation, fertilization and embedding of ovum.

M. M. Garrey, A. D. T. Govan, C. H. Hodge and R. Callander, *Obstetrics Illustrated*, 2nd edn, Churchill Livingstone, 1975, chapter 1, pp. 2–6. The Physiology of Reproduction. Clear, diagrammatic representation of ovulation, menstruation, fertilization and nidation (line drawings).

Ortho Pharmaceutical Corporation, *Understanding*, 1971, pp. 38–9. Diagrammatic representation of fertilization.

R. Rugh and L. B. Shettles, *From Conception to Birth—The Drama of Life's Beginnings*, George Allen & Unwin, 1971, pp. 4–24. Detailed text illustrated by photographs of ovulation, fertilization and cell division.

Development of the fetus and placenta
BOOKS

C. W. F. Burnett, *The Anatomy and Physiology of Obstetrics*, Faber, 1971, pp. 111–19. Clear, but elementary text describing embedding of the ovum and early development of fetus and placenta. Illustrated by line drawings.

M. M. Garrey, A. D. T. Govan, C. H. Hodge and R. Callander, *Obstetrics Illustrated*, 2nd edn, Churchill Livingstone, 1975, pp. 14–19. Development of placenta and membranes. Excellent diagrams. Elementary text. Pp. 8–13, Development of the embryo.

R. Rugh and L. B. Shettles, *From Conception to Birth—The Drama of Life's Beginnings*, George Allen & Unwin, 1971, chapter 2, pp. 25–37. Development of the placenta and fetus during the first month of life. Detailed text illustrated by extraordinary colour plates and drawings.

Menstruation
BOOKS

C. W. F. Burnett, *The Anatomy and Physiology of Obstetrics*, Faber, 1971, chapter 4, pp. 87–100. The Physiology of Menstruation. Detailed text illustrated by diagrams.

Wendy Cooper, *No Change*, Arrow Books, 1975, A lay view of the menopause.

Katherine Dalton, *The Menstrual Cycle*, Penguin, 1969. A full discussion of the physical, mental and social effects of menstruation.

D. Llewellyn-Jones, *Fundamentals of Obstetrics and Gynaecology*, vol. 2— Gynaecology, p. 58. Diagram illustrating the hormonal control of menstruation.

Ortho Pharmaceutical Corporation, *Understanding*, 1971, chapter 2, pp. 23–35. Understanding the Menstrual Cycle. The writer uses lay terminology but the information is well illustrated by clear diagrams.

B. R. Sweet and I. F. Cape, *Obstetric Care*, Nursing Modules, H.M. & M. Publishers, 1976, pp. 26–8. Brief summary of the menstrual cycle. Complementary to O.P.C.'s *Understanding*.

ARTICLES

M. M. Hall, 'A new drug for the induction of ovulation', *Nursing Mirror*, 11 Feb. 1972.

I. Mills, 'Biology of Sexuality', *Nursing Mirror*, 18 Aug. 1972.

D. Williams, 'The menopause', *Nursing Mirror*, 23 June 1972.

Chapter 3 Disorders of the uterine and menstruation
ARTICLES

E. Anstice, 'Ask any woman: menstrual problems', *Nursing Times*, 30 Nov. 1975.

J. A. Chalmers, 'Uterine fibroids', *Nursing Times*, 28 Oct. 1976. Descriptive article discussing pathology, symptomatology and management.

Jean Cope, 'The post-hysterectomy syndrome', *Nursing Times*, 14 Aug. 1976. When hysterectomy is performed for slight rather than major pathology, there is evidence that patients are more likely to suffer afterwards from severe depression.

F. G. Craddock and O. A. N. Hussein, 'A mobile cancer screening service', *Nursing Mirror*, 30 Oct. 1976. Methods used by the Women's National Cancer Control Campaign.

P. Iredale, 'Total abdominal hysterectomy and bilateral salpingo-oöphorectomy', Nursing Care Study, *Nursing Times*, 22 July 1976.

F. A. Langley, 'Pre-malignancy in gynaecology', *Nursing Mirror*, 29 Jan. 1976. Discussion of the special type of histological changes in the tissue that may be followed by invasive tumour.

I. Martin, 'Psychiatric aspects of menstrual disorder', *Nursing Times*, 13 Nov. 1975.

A. T. Mennie and C. Long, 'Pain relief for gynaecological caesium removal', *Nursing Times*, 25 Sept. 1975. Introducing the use of Entonox when the source is being removed at the end of treatment.

J. R. Newton and C. Vaughan Williams, 'Menstrual disorders', *Nursing Mirror*, 30 Jan. 1975.

Josephine Williamson, 'Carcinoma of the body of the uterus', *Nursing Times*, 27 May 1976. Helpful descriptive article of this disease.

B. E. P. Wookey, 'Well women clinic in group practice', *Nursing Mirror*, 4 Feb. 1972.

Chapter 4 Disorders of the ovary and oviducts
Infertility
BOOKS

B. Law, *Woman and her Fertility*, April 1972.

J. G. Lewis, *The Endocrine System*, Penguin Library of Nursing, Penguin Education, 1973, chapter 8, pp. 180–3. Brief description of the physiological causes and some suggested methods of treatment.

D. Llewellyn-Jones, *Fundamentals of Obstetrics and Gynaecology*, vol. 2 – Gynaecology, Faber, 1975, chapter 10. Infertility.

R. Newill, *Infertile Marriage*, Penguin Handbooks, 1974. Describes in detail the physical causes and treatments for infertility and subfertility both in men and women. In addition, the author deals fully with the psychological implications and discusses miscarriage and the 'alternatives' of adoption and artificial insemination.

ARTICLES

C. N. Hudson, 'Cancer of the ovary', *Nursing Mirror*, 6 April 1973.

Cicely Saunders, *Care of the Dying*, Nursing Times Publications, 1976.

S. E. Smith, 'Drugs and cancer: how drugs act', *Nursing Times*, 27 Nov. 1975.

R. W. Taylor, 'Infertility—the role of the fallopian tubes', *Nursing Mirror*, vol. 133, 3 Sept. 1971, pp. 22–3.

K. Westbrook, 'Coping with relatives', *Nursing Mirror*, 2 June 1972.

Chapter 5 Disorders of the vagina and vulva
BOOK

R. S. Morton, *Venereal Diseases*, Pelican Publications, 1972. Frank and sober study of syphilis, gonorrhoea and other diseases commonly transmitted during sexual intercourse.

ARTICLES

A. Akpason, 'Vesico-vaginal fistula', Nursing Care Study, *Nursing Mirror*, Sept. 1972.

J. Barnes, 'Backache in women', *Nursing Mirror*, 31 March 1975.

A. P. Bentall, 'Carcinoma of the vulva', *Nursing Mirror*, 27 Feb. 1975.

W. K. Bernfield, 'Sexually transmitted diseases', *Nursing Mirror*, 27 Dec. 1972.

G. M. Besser, 'Hirsutes', *Nursing Mirror*, 5 May 1972.

T. Brown, 'Trichomonas vaginilis', *Nursing Mirror*, 27 March 1975.

C. N. Hudson, 'Obstetric fistulae', *Nursing Mirror*, 18 May 1970.

C. N. Hudson, 'Irritation of the vulva', *Nursing Mirror*, 19 May 1972.

J. S. Tomkinson, 'Carcinoma of the vulva', *Nursing Times*, 3 June 1976. Descriptive article discussing differential diagnosis treatment and progress.

Chapter 6 Painful conditions of the female genitalia
BOOKS

J. Chalmers, *Endometriosis*, Butterworth, 1975.

A. J. Harding Rains, V. Rains and M. Mackenzie, *Urgencies and Emergencies for Nurses*, English University Press, 1965. Written to help both general and specialist nursing staff when faced with a wide range of emergencies.

ARTICLES

J. Willocks, 'Recognising ectopic pregnancy despite deceptive symptoms', *Modern Medicine*, Sept. 1976.

Chapter 7 Prolapse and displacements
ARTICLES

S. Balch and C. N. Hudson, 'Prolapse', (three articles), *Nursing Times*, 26 Aug., 2 Sept. and 9 Sept. 1966.

J. P. Blandy, 'Catheterization', *Nursing Mirror*, 2 June 1972.

'Incontinence', Symposium published by Nursing Times Publications, 1976.

C. M. Lade, 'Marsupial pants for urinary incontinence', *Nursing Mirror*, 18 Aug. 1972.

Jane Stronge, 'Infection of the urinary tract associated with catheters', *Nursing Times*, 18 March 1972.

S. G. Tuffill, 'Urinary diversion', *Nursing Mirror*, 14 Jan. 1972.

Chapter 8 Disorders of pregnancy
Diseases of the trophoblast
BOOKS

I. Donald, *Practical Obstetric Problems*, 4th edn, Lloyd-Luke, 1969, pp. 64–78. Describes in detail the symptoms diagnosis and management of hydatidiform mole and choriocarcinoma.

D. Llewellyn-Jones, *Fundamentals of Obstetrics and Gynaecology*, vol. 2 – Gynaecology, 4th edn, Faber, 1975, chapter 20, pp. 192–200. A clear classification of benign and malignant tumours of the trophoblast illustrated by photographs. The text describes diagnosis, management and prognosis of trophoblastic disease.

M. Myles, *Textbook for Midwives*, 8th edn, Churchill Livingstone, 1975, pp. 141–2. A brief summary of signs, symptoms and treatment. Complementary to the above.

Ectopic gestation
BOOK

D. Llewellyn-Jones, *Fundamentals of Obstetrics and Gynaecology*, vol. 2 – Gynaecology, 4th edn, Faber, 1975, chapter 22, pp. 209–14. Concise summary of the aetiology, pathology and management of ectopic gestation, with clear diagrammatic representation.

ARTICLES

Nursing Times, 2 May 1974, pp. 669–71. Nursing Care Study of a patient who conceived following treatment for infertility. Examination revealed one intra-uterine pregnancy and one tubal pregnancy. The former resulted in a spontaneous abortion and the latter was dealt with by surgical intervention.

T. G. Nash, 'Tubal Pregnancy and other sites', *Nursing Times*, 17 Oct. 1974 pp. 1623–4. Illustrated by photographs.

F. C. R. Picton, 'Ectopic gestation', *Nursing Times*, 2 May 1974, pp. 672–3. A comprehensive article based on the aetiology, diagnosis treatment and management of ectopic gestation. A clear diagram of the uterus and adenexa illustrates the main sites of ectopic pregnancy.

Report on Confidential Enquiries into Maternal Deaths in England and Wales, 1970–72, published by H.M.S.O., 1975. Ectopic pregnancy. Statistical information relating to the mortality associated with ectopic pregnancy and avoidable factors.

Chapter 8
Abortion
BOOKS

Sir Stanely G. Clayton, D. Fraser and T. L. T. Lewis (Eds.), *Obstetrics by Ten Teachers,* Arnold, 1972, chapter 17, pp. 173–90. Comprehensive study of the causes of abortion, clinical varieties and treatment.

R. F. F. Gardner, *Abortion—The Personal Dilemma,* Paternoster Press, 1972. Preface by John Stallworthy. This book examines the moral, ethical, religious, physical and mental issues involved in this emotive subject.

Report on Confidential Enquiries into Maternal Deaths in England and Wales, 1970–72, published by Her Majesty's Stationery Office, London, 1975, chapter 5, pp. 39–49. This report covers the first complete triennium during which the Abortion Act (1967) has been operative. As in the last four reports, abortion remains the largest single cause of maternal death, and this report presents important statistical evidence relating to the mortality associated with spontaneous, legal and illegal abortion.

ARTICLES

M. Barnett, 'Socio-economic factors affecting contraception', *Nursing Times,* 25 Nov. 1976.

John Beazley, 'The prostaglandins', *Nursing Times,* 18 Nov. 1976. Discussion of their chemical potential and their broad clinical application not only in induction of term labour and termination of pregnancy.

E. R. Bickerstaff, 'Neurological complications of the pill', *Nursing Mirror,* 19 May 1972.

R. Binning, 'Abortion—on demand or request?', *World Medicine,* 28 July 1976.

C. Brewer, 'Mortal coils. Legal paradoxes of post conceptive contraception', *World Medicine,* 2 June 1976.

Committee on Safety of Medicines Report, 'Cancer and the pill', *Nursing Mirror,* 17 Nov. 1972.

Jean Dewhurst and A. Weeks, 'Occult manifestation of septic abortion', *Nursing Mirror*, 29 April 1976.

J. O. Greenhalf, 'Termination of a mid-trimester pregnancy', *Nursing Mirror*, vol. 134, 2 June 1972, pp. 34–6. Methods of termination and results.

J. Marshall, 'Methods of contraception', *Nursing Mirror*, 27 April 1975.

D. E. Morris, 'Chorimepithelioma', Nursing Care Study, *Nursing Mirror*, 16 June 1972.

'Oral contraceptives', a memorandum to the D.H.S.S. from the Patients Association, *Nursing Times*, 23 Oct. 1975. Working party report on whether oral contraceptives should be available without prescription and whether specially trained nurses and midwives should be allowed to prescribe them.

'Risk of pelvic infection associated with intra uterine devices', *British Medical Journal*, 25 Sept. 1976.

A. B. Sclare, 'Termination of pregnancy—the nurse's attitude', *Nursing Mirror*, 16 Jan. 1975.

Upjohn. The use of Prostaglandins E_2 and F_2 alpha in Obstetrics and Gynaecology. Published following the Symposium sponsored by Upjohn. A series of papers on the use of prostaglandins for mid-trimester termination.

Saffron Whitehead, 'New trends in contraception', *Nursing Times*, 25 Nov. 1976.

C. Young, 'Termination of pregnancy', *British Journal of Hospital Medicine*, Aug. 1976. Description of methods, complications and after care.

Index